'The book is part of the extremely topical and socially important issues relating to the body image in eating disorders in the context of psychological diagnosis and therapy. Certainly, this monograph will find an audience among patients with eating disorders and their families, as well as specialists in many professions (including psychologists, doctors, teachers, psychotherapists), as well as students in the field of medical, psychological, pedagogical or people who want to specialize in psychotherapy for people with eating disorders, both children, adolescents and adults.'

Mariola Bidzan, *Professor, Department of Clinical and Health Psychology, University of Gdansk, Poland*

'*Body Image in Eating Disorders* is a valuable publication, especially for theorists and researchers of body image phenomena and eating disorders, as well as for psychotherapists. I consider the results of the author's research extremely valuable for understanding non-constructive behaviors towards the body and eating, especially in the adolescent and young adult population.'

Beata Ziółkowska, *Professor, Department of Psychology, Kazimierz Wielki University, Bydgoszcz, Poland*

Body Image in Eating Disorders

Body Image in Eating Disorders explores issues relating to the prevention, clinical diagnosis, and psychological treatment of distortions of body image in eating disorders. It presents a multifactorial model of indicators for diagnosis and treatment, considering psychological, sociocultural, and family indicators.

Based on original empirical research with women and girls suffering from eating disorders, the book draws attention to limitations and dilemmas related to psychological diagnosis and treatment of people with eating disorders including anorexia readiness syndrome, bulimia, and bigorexia. The book proposes an integrative psychodynamic approach to the diagnosis and treatment of body image disorders and presents case studies illustrating examples of application of integration of psychodynamic therapy and psychodrama in psychological treatment of young people suffering from eating disorders. It considers risk factors including abnormal body image for the development of eating disorders and argues that psychological diagnosis of the body image is an important factor in determining the right direction of psychological treatment for people with eating disorders.

Drawing on theoretical foundations and evidence-based clinical practice, the book will be of great interest to researchers, academics, and students in the fields of clinical and applied psychology, mental health, and specialists in eating disorders.

Bernadetta Izydorczyk is a professor at the Institute of Psychology, Faculty of Philosophy of the Jagiellonian University in Krakow.

Advances in Mental Health Research series

Body Image in Eating Disorders

Clinical Diagnosis and Integrative Approach to Psychological Treatment

Bernadetta Izydorczyk

Routledge
Taylor & Francis Group

LONDON AND NEW YORK

First published 2022
by Routledge
2 Park Square, Milton Park, Abingdon, Oxon OX14 4RN

and by Routledge
605 Third Avenue, New York, NY 10158

Routledge is an imprint of the Taylor & Francis Group, an informa business

British Library Cataloguing-in-Publication Data
A catalogue record for this book is available from the British Library

Library of Congress Cataloging-in-Publication Data
A catalog record has been requested for this book

ISBN: 978-1-032-13862-6 (hbk)
ISBN: 978-1-032-16948-4 (pbk)
ISBN: 978-1-003-25108-8 (ebk)

DOI: 10.4324/9781003251088

Typeset in Times New Roman
by MPS Limited, Dehradun

Contents

Figures

Tables

Acknowledgments

The open access license fee of the publication was funded by the Priority Research Area Society of the Future under the program "Excellence Initiative – Research University" at the Jagiellonian University in Krakow.

Introduction

This book is the result of the author's many years of theoretical and empirical experience in her clinical practice with diagnosis and psychotherapy of eating disorders. As a clinical psychologist, psychotherapist, and supervisor, in taking up the challenge of developing guidelines for clinical psychological diagnosis of body image in patients with eating disorders, the author referred to the principles of evidence-based practice. This book is addressed to a wide audience: psychology and pedagogy students, psychologists, psychotherapists, psychiatrists, and other specialists who, in their daily practice, increasingly struggle with problems related to the diagnosis and psychological support for patients with eating disorders.

This book is devoted to very important issues in prevention, clinical diagnosis, and psychological treatment of body image distortions in eating disorders. The directions of the process and the criteria of psychological diagnosis of body image presented in this book were developed on the basis of psychodynamic theory, which has been well-established in the scientific literature for many years. The author also refers to many years of own research carried out in this paradigm, the core of which comprised the search for and empirical verification of the importance of the personality structure for the development of body image distortions in patients with eating disorders exhibiting tendencies toward anorexic, bulimic, and bigorexic anti-health behaviors. The contents of the individual chapters of this book contribute to the clinical and scientific knowledge in the field of prevention, diagnosis, and psychological treatment of body image distortions in patients with eating disorders, additionally taking into account the advantages and limitations of the proposed diagnostic criteria and therapeutic indications.

Chapter 1 presents contemporary theoretical and empirical reflections on:

- the definition of body image – the structure of the body Self as a predictor of eating behaviors in the context of sociocultural and technological changes;
- the specificity and importance of the body as a significant object in the process of psychological diagnosis and psychotherapy;
- the psychosocial functions of food in shaping body image.

DOI: 10.4324/9781003251088-101

Regardless of the diversity of definitions of body image, the psychological diagnosis of cognitive and emotional body image distortions and behaviors toward the body in eating disorders require reference to evidence-based practice in medicine and clinical psychology. This involves taking into account the empirical measurement of multiple psychosocial variables outlined in this book in relation to the results of the author's own research.

In Chapter 2, the author indicates the importance of (a) family types and family/sociocultural myths about body image and food as well as (b) patterns of emotional attachment as predictors of body image distortions in patients with eating disorders. The chapter summarizes the results of the author's research on psychological and sociocultural body image profiles in young, healthy Polish women and men as predictors of the development of anorexic readiness, bulimia, and bigorexia (in men). The author presents the results of statistical analyses indicating three specific female and three specific male psychological and sociocultural body image profiles.

Chapter 3 presents psychological data documenting the importance of various psychological traumas and their significant symptoms in the process of diagnosing body image distortions in eating disorders. The author presents this issue in the context of her own research on women with anorexia, bulimia, and binge eating disorder.

Chapter 4 focuses on the elements and characteristics of diagnosis of eating disorders (based on previous results, including the author's own research), including the so-called anorexic readiness and bigorexia indicators. The author presents her own study of a sample of adolescent girls and young women with anorexia and bulimia, examining their psychological profiles and dispositions.

Chapter 5 describes the indicators for clinical diagnosis of the personality structure in the context of structure-specific body image features among patients with eating disorders. Based on the theory of object relations and Kernberg's model of personality structure organization, the author presents the justification for and description of diagnostic indicators of personality structures (neurotic, borderline, and psychotic) in the context of diagnosing specific body image features.

Chapter 6 proposes an integrative approach to the psychological treatment of body image distortions in eating disorders. The author points to nonspecific and specific therapeutic factors and attempts to integrate the psychodynamic, behavioral, and psychodrama approaches. These theoretical considerations are presented in light of clinical case descriptions of people with eating disorders undergoing psychodynamic (group or individual) psychotherapy with simultaneously implemented elements of cognitive-behavioral and psychodrama techniques to treat body image distortions.

Chapter 7 presents the psychological justification for and description of the psychodrama and in the individual and group therapies, in which the protagonists are patients with eating disorders. The patients usually focus on the topics of hatred of the body and conflicts around eating. Psychodrama techniques can significantly accelerate the process of working through and/ or bypassing resistance when identifying emotional and cognitive body image distortions. When a patient during psychological therapy plays psychodrama roles connected with body image and eating disorders symptoms, hence he has a bigger chance to quickly overcome the phenomenon of universal resistance.

Chapter 8 presents a summary of data from the literature and clinical practice on the basic psychosocial factors which are important from the perspective of carrying out a psychological diagnosis of body image distortions among patients suffering from various types of eating disorders. Specifying the role of particular psychological and social (as well as sociocultural) factors in shaping body image and various related behaviors is significant from the point of view of treatment planning with eating disorder patients.

In sum, the overarching goal of this book is to present important diagnostic and therapeutic factors for body image distortions, as indicated by theoreticians and documented in the author's research project, to psychologists, psychotherapists, psychiatrists, and other mental health professionals as well as students of psychology and other social sciences and medical fields.

1 The phenomenon of body image: a psychological perspective

Chapter 1 presents the theoretical and empirical arguments for the importance of taking a multidimensional perspective on defining the phenomenon of body image in the process of psychological diagnosis of body image distortions as well as the process of psychotherapy of eating disorders. The multi-factor model of psychosocial risk factors for body image distortions and anti-health eating behaviors (restrictive, compulsive, and bulimic) presented in Chapter 1 is in line with the principles of evidence-based practice, which is necessary for its use in treatment of eating disorders.

Body image: a predictor of anti-health behaviors toward eating

During literature reviews and analyses of clinical experiences of psychologists and other specialists cooperating in the process of treating eating disorders, it should be assumed that regardless of the adopted theoretical paradigm (psychoanalytical, cognitive-behavioral, and sociocultural), specific and nonspecific eating disorders in adolescents and adults are disorders characterized by ambiguity, complex determinants and mechanisms of development, and diverse self-destructive (restrictive, bulimic, and compulsive) behaviors toward eating and one's own body (Cash & Pruzinsky, 2004; Izydorczyk, 2015; Józefik, 2008, 2014). The body image in eating disorders is also complex and multifaceted. Most of its definitions, both in cognitive, psychoanalytical, and sociocultural theories, highlight its emotional (satisfaction/dissatisfaction with appearance and weight), cognitive (perception, estimation of its dimensions, schema regarding one's own body and appearance), and behavioral (the behaviors toward the body) aspects (Cash, 2004, 2012; Schier, 2010; Thompson & Smolak, 2001). Body image is a mental structure describing the experience of the individual's internal world in relation to the external (social, i.e., shared with other people) environment, simultaneously taking into account its emotional background which develops across the lifespan through relations with others.

Body image is an element of the personality structure of the body Self, and thus a component of the personality structure of the Self (Higgins, 1987). According to Higgins' self-discrepancy theory, people strive to reduce

DOI: 10.4324/9781003251088-1

the differences (discrepancies) between how they perceive themselves (actual Self) and what they would like to be (ideal Self) or should be (ought Self, Higgins 1987). The discrepancy between the actual Self and another specific type of Self-standard (e.g., the ideal Self) is reflected in the content of cognitive schemas indicating an unfavorable (negative) psychological situation for the person which has emotional and motivational consequences for behaviors toward the body and eating (Cash & Pruzinsky, 2004; Izydorczyk, 2015a; Thompson & Smolak, 2001).

In cognitive theories, an important factor explaining the formation of body image is the sociocultural influence and body image standards promoted in the culture of westernization (Izydorczyk & Sitnik-Warchulska, 2018; Izydorczyk et al., 2020). The nature and strength of the attitudes adopted by a person toward the assimilation of sociocultural standards of an ideal body influence his undertaking of pro- or anti-health behaviors in relation to his body and eating.

In the theory of body objectification, Fredrickson and Roberts (1997) emphasize the importance of self-sexualization, in which girls and young women treat their bodies – themselves – as sexual objects. From the perspective of the psychoanalytical–psychodynamic paradigm, body image is an element of the personality structure of the Self, called the body Self (Krueger, 2002a, 2002b; Sakson-Obada, 2008). The structure of the body Self and the psychological quality of experiencing the body (in perception, thoughts, and emotions) are influenced by autobiographical experiences (especially during childhood). Trauma theories prove that trauma, sexual violence, and violations of personal boundaries, especially in childhood, cause developmental distortions in experiencing one's body and in building close, emotional relationships with others in the future (Izydorczyk, 2017a; Krystal, 2000; Madowitz et al., 2015; McDougall, 2014; Sakson-Obada, 2008, 2009a, 2009b).

The psychodynamic approach and attachment theory not only focus on the cognitive and emotional assessment of the external body (body image), but also on learning about oneself through the body, that is, the experience of body functions, control of incoming stimuli and emotions as well as acceptance of one's psychosexual identity (Krueger, 2002a, 2002b; Sakson-Obada, 2009b; Skrzypska & Suchańska, 2011). Summarizing the above-mentioned review of the basic claims of psychological theories concerning body image, it is worth pointing to the validity of the statement that it is impossible to treat patients with eating disorders without targeting the psychological mechanisms of body image distortions.

Anorexia and bulimia nervosa or binge eating disorder are disorders in which both the body and the mental Self are simultaneously affected (Józefik, 2008; Józefik et al., 2010; Krueger, 2002a, 2002b; McDougall, 2014). At each stage of treatment of various types of eating disorders, addressing both the patients' somatic health and mental well-being is necessary to re-establish their biopsychosocial balance (Domaradzki, 2013; World

Health Organization, 2018). Patients with eating disorders can exhibit various levels of personality structure pathology: from the neurotic to the borderline and psychotic (Gabbard, 2015). The level of dysfunction in the personality structure also determines the direction and form of (medical and psychotherapeutic) interventions in the course of the entire treatment process (Clarkin et al., 2013; Gabbard, 2015). In order to provide comprehensive treatment, apart from examining the personality structure, which may present various levels of destabilization, it is also worth to conduct a psychological diagnosis of various body image distortions.

Depending on the destabilization of the personality structure and individual life history (especially the history of psychological traumas) patients may present with various cognitive deficits (or even defects) concerning the perception of the body and its individual parts, negative thoughts and emotions about body image, as well as interoceptive deficits related to the differentiation of various stimuli from the body (Garner, 2004; Izydorczyk, 2011; 2013a, 2013b, 2015). Psychosomatic theories and their application in clinical practice indicate that people who are unaware of the frustration of their important emotional needs, internal conflicts, and emotional deficits often experience somatic symptoms – their bodies suffer (McDougall, 2014; Sakson-Obada, 2008, 2009a, 2009b; Schier, 2010). The somatic symptom is a specific symbol of unconscious and highly diversified internal conflict (Krueger, 2002a, 2002b; McDougall, 2014; Schier, 2010).

When making a psychological diagnosis of the mechanisms underlying the symptoms of anorexia and bulimia, it is worth reflecting on the symbolic functions of restrictive and/or compulsive (bulimic) eating behaviors. Such destructive behaviors as restrictive, debilitating attempts to lose weight, fasting, provoking vomiting, and other forms of purging are often puzzling in their purpose. Why does the patient dislike their body and devalue it in such unfavorable, unhealthy ways? There are many questions, and they all center around the body. The body is subject to restrictive or impulsive actions that harm life and health, and it must be taken into account both in the process of diagnosis and treatment.

A comprehensive (medical, psychotherapeutic, and dietary) treatment process of patients with eating disorders always takes into account multidirectional interactions, which, depending on the adopted therapeutic paradigm, include interventions focused on restoring health. This also means compensating for disturbances in the cognitive and emotional experience of body image. In the process of treatment of body image distortions, patients with anorexia, bulimia, or binge eating disorder often require support in recognizing and eliminating/reducing these distortions and in shaping healthy eating behaviors (Cash & Pruzinsky, 2004; Izydorczyk, 2015; Vartanian et al., 2018; Wertheim et al., 2004). Psychotherapeutic treatment of emotional and cognitive body image distortions is one of the most important aspects of treating patients with various types of eating disorders. It utilizes specific, professional diagnostic measures in order to completely remove or reduce the symptoms of eating disorders.

Psychotherapy of eating disorders, including body image distortions, should be multidirectional and dependent on the patient's current health condition and needs (in a situation of physical exhaustion, it will be much more limited than when the patients' psychophysical well-being is better and their condition is no longer life-threatening). The psychological diagnosis of the perception and thoughts and negative emotions about body image is a significant complement to the diagnosis of a specific personality structure and a psychological profile (especially intense emotional dysregulation, fear, excessive perfectionism, impulsivity, low self-esteem, lack of self-confidence, distrust and uncertainty in emotional relationships; Izydorczyk, 2011, 2013a, 2013b, 2015; Mikołajczyk & Samochowiec, 2004a, 2004b). Such a comprehensive psychological diagnosis is needed to determine the appropriate psychotherapeutic treatment for patients with eating disorders presenting a diverse spectrum of destructive behaviors toward the body and eating.

The dominant influence of sociocultural factors and psychosocial determinants on the relationship between unfinished separation and individuation in adolescents, the formation of body image, and the escalation of destructive behavior toward the body (based on the drive for thinness and emotional dissatisfaction) indicates a different direction of psychotherapy (often with the use of family therapy) than situations where adult patients experience body image distortions and simultaneously present a destabilization of the personality structure at the borderline or psychotic level (Gabbard, 2015; Izydorczyk, 2010; 2015, 2017b). The dominance of perfectionism or impulsivity together with low self-esteem and distrust in interpersonal relationships (i.e., difficulties in building an emotional bond) may significantly hinder the course of the entire therapeutic process, but also determine the specificity of therapeutic interventions aimed at the body. A review of definitions of body image in psychology shows their ambiguity and varied etiology as well as the differences of diagnosing specific and nonspecific eating disorders in the ICD-10 (World Health Organization, 1993) and DSM-V (American Psychiatric Association, 2013) medical classifications (Garner, 2004). Psychiatric diagnosis is not a sufficient criterion for diagnosing the pathogenesis of eating disorders. It requires a multifactorial approach to neurobiological and psychosocial causes showing the relationship between mental disorders and eating disorders, for example, the occurrence of symptoms of psychological anorexia (Södersten et al., 2019). For this reason, a clinical psychological diagnosis including the multifactorial determinants of eating behaviors becomes necessary to determine the direction of treatment and psychotherapy (Södersten et al., 2019).

The psychological profiles of patients with eating disorders and the diagnostic criteria for anorexia and bulimia nervosa present in the ICD-10 (World Health Organization, 1993), ICD-11 (World Health Organization,

2018), and DSM-V (American Psychiatric Association, 2013) emphasize the etiological importance of the relationship between cognitive body image distortions, fear of gaining weight (fat phobia), restrictive eating behaviors (diets), excessive physical activity, and impulsive (bulimic) behaviors consisting in purging the body without existing health indications (e.g., inducing vomiting; Vartanian et al., 2018; Wertheim et al., 2004). Both theorists and researchers have confirmed the multifactorial model of the determinants of restrictive and impulsive (bulimic) eating behaviors, emphasizing the mediating role of body image distortions and dissatisfaction in their formation (Terhoeven et al., 2020; Vartanian et al., 2018; Wertheim et al., 2004). The mediating role of body image is consistent with the multifactorial cognitive models of the development of body dissatisfaction (Cash & Smolak, 2011) and its role in eating behaviors (Wertheim Thompson 2004; Rodgers et al., 2020; Vartanian et al., 2018; Wertheim et al., 2004). According to the basic assumptions of contemporary models, the determinants of the relationship between body image (satisfaction/dissatisfaction) and the development of risky (restrictive, impulsive, and bulimic) eating behaviors is multifactorial in nature (Vartanian et al., 2018). Assuming the necessity to exclude a biological basis of the dysfunctional relationship between body image and eating disorders for the purpose of medical diagnosis, it is worth pointing out that, regardless the different definitions of body image, the psychological diagnosis of cognitive and emotional body image distortions and behaviors toward the body in eating disorders requires reference to evidence-based practice, and thus, requires measuring a multivariate set of psychosocial variables (Fig. 1.1).

This model comprises the scientifically documented clinical psychological diagnosis of risky behaviors toward the body and eating. It indicates the need to account for specific risk factors (apart from age, adolescence and young adulthood, and female gender), especially ones affecting self-esteem (including body esteem), and provoking appearance-related fears (the discrepancy between the ideal and the actual body mass index, BMI). They include (a) irregularities in the functioning of the generational family (the pattern of emotional bonds, boundary-setting, generational messages, and family myths, including ones about eating habits, functions of eating, and body image), (b) psychological trauma, and (c) pressure and internalization of existing sociocultural body image standards (Cash & Pruzinsky, 2004; Cash & Smolak, 2011; Józefik et al., 2002; Izydorczyk, 2015). The specificity of the development of eating behaviors may also be influenced by the individual personality structure, in particular the body Self and the Self concept.

Dissatisfaction with body image and appearance-related fears influenced by the above factors result in engaging in restrictive, impulsive, and/or bulimic risky eating behaviors. Before presenting the individual elements of the psychological diagnosis in the model, the main points confirming the importance of experiencing the patient's and the therapist's bodies as entities remaining together in the entire therapeutic process are presented.

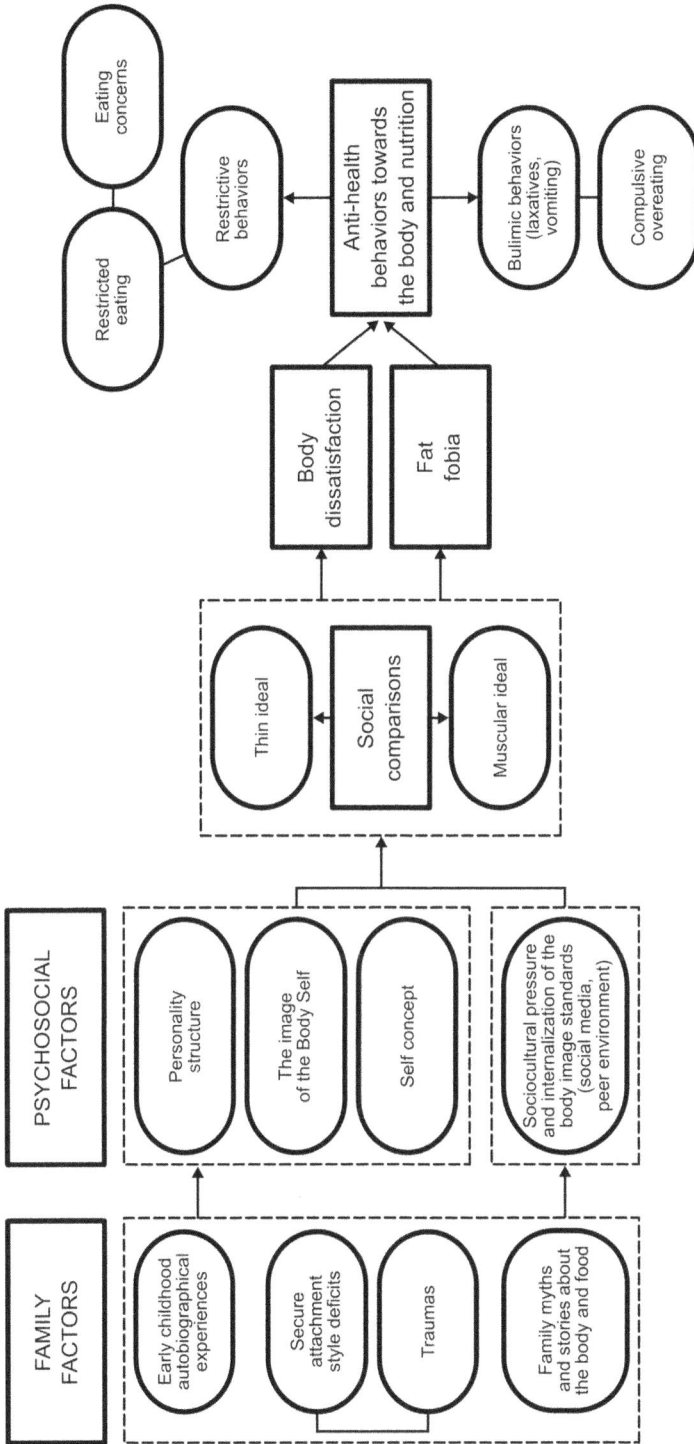

Figure 1.1 The multi-factor model of psychosocial risk factors for the development of anti-health eating behaviors (own elaboration).

The body as a subject in the process of psychological diagnosis and psychotherapy

From birth, humans are endowed with organs and senses that help explore the world. Knowledge about the world is bodyoriented. The body first "understands" the world, distinguishing its elements and acting in such a way as to achieve further developmental goals. In phenomenological terms, the body is not just a causal mechanism, but an "intentional" whole that is always directed toward an object in the world (Lemma, 2014, 2016; McDougall, 2014; Sakson-Obada, 2008, Schier, 2010). Psychological diagnosis and therapy are thus an "embodied process" – an encounter between two minds and bodies, that of the psychologist and his patient. As indicated by developmental and clinical psychology literature and psychosomatic theories, the body perceives through its senses and identifies emotions and sensations. The body is an anchor in the present, constituting the border between the present and the past, allowing for a kind of "escape" from the past, for example, traumatic events (Izydorczyk, 2017a; Józefik, 2008; Sakson-Obada, 2009a, 2009b). The early childhood pattern of the child's emotional bond with the mother, her ability to rhythmically tune in to the child (reflecting feelings in the eyes, movements, gestures, touch, words, and expressions) is a psychological material that connects the mother and the infant (projective identification) and gives boundaries to the mental structure. This is the basis for creating a connection between the mind and the *psyche* (Krueger, 2002b; McDougall, 2014).

The level of mental development and embodied experience of the body of the eating disorder patient becomes an important element of psychological and psychotherapeutic diagnosis. From the perspective of human psychological development described in this way, diagnosis and psychological therapy should be understood as a way of constructing meaning through the meeting of the patient's and the therapist's minds and bodies. This meeting provides the therapist with significant clues about the patient's inner world. The sensations flowing from the body and experienced physically and mentally by the therapist in contact with the patient are an important element supporting both the diagnosis and psychological therapy of eating disorders. From the perspective of therapy in the psychodynamic approach and the operation of unconscious psychological mechanisms of projection and transference/countertransference, the patients' specific reaction to the psychologist in the real therapeutic relationship also unconsciously reflects their pattern of relationship with the main caregiver in early childhood (reflected through emotional and cognitive functioning; Glickauf-Hughes & Wells, 1997; Józefik, 2008; Józefik et al., 2010; Krueger, 2002a).

Object relation theories indicate the importance of internalized interpersonal relationships and their influence on behavior throughout the lifespan. They particularly focus on childhood internalization of early interaction patterns with parents or caregivers (Clarkin et al., 2013; Gabbard, 2015;

Glickauf-Hughes & Wells, 1997; Izydorczyk, 2010; Krueger, 2002a, 2002b; McWilliams, 2014). The relationship matrix of the child with the social environment consists of an image of itself and an internalized objects – representations of the child's experiences in relation with its caregivers (especially the parents). The diagnosis of this internal image allows to better understand and recognize the patients' interpersonal behaviors and modify their internal character structure (representations of objects, oneself, and the emotional world). From the beginning of the diagnostic and/or therapeutic contact, the patients' emotional pattern of their relationship with the caregiver in childhood is projected onto the doctor, psychologist, or psychotherapist. The patients and their body can directly react to the contact with the therapist and their body with a rich repertoire of feelings, from pain, suffering, and anger, to pleasure, love, and joy, which are felt on the physical level, creating a unique, personal inner world (Clarkin et al., 2013; Glickauf-Hughes & Wells, 1997; Lemma, 2014; McDougall, 2014). The body is an instrument of physical processes, an instrument that can hear, see, touch, and smell the surrounding world. It is a subject that reacts to the diagnostic and therapeutic relationship depending on its current psychophysical state: from cachexia to stabilized somatic functioning (Lemma, 2016; McDougall, 2014).

The patients' bodily reactions to the therapeutic relationship allow for refining the diagnosis of their psychological functioning. In many situations of the patient's physical exhaustion (heart rhythm disturbances, insufficient body weight), immediate measures must be taken to compensate for nutritional deficiencies because they are a direct threat to the patient's life. Such patients usually require inpatient treatment. In such cases, the diagnostic and psychotherapeutic work to make the patient aware of the unconscious internal conflicts and mechanisms underlying the eating disorder becomes meaningless. A physically exhausted person is unable to use his emotional resources to change his mental functioning. Therefore, making a decision about hospitalization, where the patient is under constant care and supervision, is the basic therapeutic intervention saving the patient's body and life (Izydorczyk, 2015; Józefik et al., 2002).

Psychological support in regulating the patients' behaviors toward their body is required in this situation. However, this is not always accepted by the patient. It often arouses resistance and negation of the doctor/therapist's position. For example, due to many pathological psychological mechanisms (denial, primitive idealization, splitting, projective identification, rationalization, intellectualization), patients with anorexia block (cut off) their emotional experience of the body and cognitively distort (through schemas and perception) its image. They experience their body differently than the psychologist, therapist, or doctor does. Identification with the disease and the distortions taking place in the mental world do not allow the patients to realistically assess their life-threatening and destructive attitude toward their body. Sometimes, despite the patient's protests, hospitalization is the only correct choice at a later stage of the treatment (Izydorczyk, 2017b; Józefik et al., 2002).

Therefore, it is worth assuming from the very beginning of the diagnosis process and treatment of eating disorders that the body is a sensitive instrument in the therapeutic relationship that also has the ability to adjust to the mental functioning of a person in a relationship with another human being. The body is an important subject of therapeutic influence during treatment, and the treatment itself should be multidirectional and include specialist forms of medical, psychotherapeutic, and dietary interactions adapted to the current stage of the disorder's development.

Psychosocial functions of food *versus* body image

The attitude toward food is defined in the literature as a multidimensional construct regulating cognitive and affective processes as well as behaviors related to eating and nutrition. The affective, cognitive, and behavioral attitude toward food and eating may be positive (adaptive eating habits, eating is a source of pleasure) or negative (disorders of control overeating, eating does not satisfy hunger and biopsychosocial health needs), as in the case of of anorexia, bulimia, and binge eating disorder, or, increasingly often, orthorexia and bigorexia.

Attitudes toward food are extremely resistant to change because they are part of the Self structure. Food satisfies biological and mental needs. Through its sociocultural functions, it also determines the individual sense of identity. The part of the personality that determines the sense of identity is the structure of the Self, including the body Self (Izydorczyk, 2015; Krueger, 2002a, 2002b; Sakson-Obada, 2008). Hence, it can be assumed that the specificity of the psychosocial functions of eating and the symbolic meaning of food (nourishment) for the understanding of unconscious internal conflicts of patients with eating disorders are related to the structure of the body Self (body image) as an integral part of the personality structure. This relationship is presented in detail in Chapter 5. Niewiadomska et al. (2005) divided the functions of food into biological, psychological, worldview-related, social, cultural, and economic functions (Fig. 1.2).

The biological function of food has been defined as "the body's absorption of substances from the external environment, constituting a material for building and restoring body components, and a source of energy" (Encyklopedia PWN, 2018). Such an understanding assigns food a physiological function that guarantees survival and development in the biological sense. On the other hand, the psychosocial functions of food are all extra-biological functions that are fulfilled by personal food choices, for example, the emotional (transmitter for emotions) or social function (transmitter of interpersonal relations), building/maintaining relationships, maintaining control, expressing views, reinforcing myths, and giving punishments/rewards (Józefik, 2014; Niewiadomska et al, 2005).

In western cultures, food is also associated with patterns of body image attractiveness. Regulation of eating strengthens the sense of agency, which is often important in the etiology of eating disorders. People who are deprived of influence in their own lives through an overly oppressive upbringing may

Biological functions	→	Drawing netrients which help maintain the body life processes
Psychological functions	→	Satisfying various mental needs (e.g. love, security, recognition)
Worldview functions	→	Food selection and preparation as an expression of beliefs or religion
Social functions	→	Establishing and maintaining interpersonal relations
Cultural functions	→	Culinary arts, Food aesthetics, Food obtaining as a progress in the civiliztion development
Economic functions	→	A product intended for advertising, sale and consumption

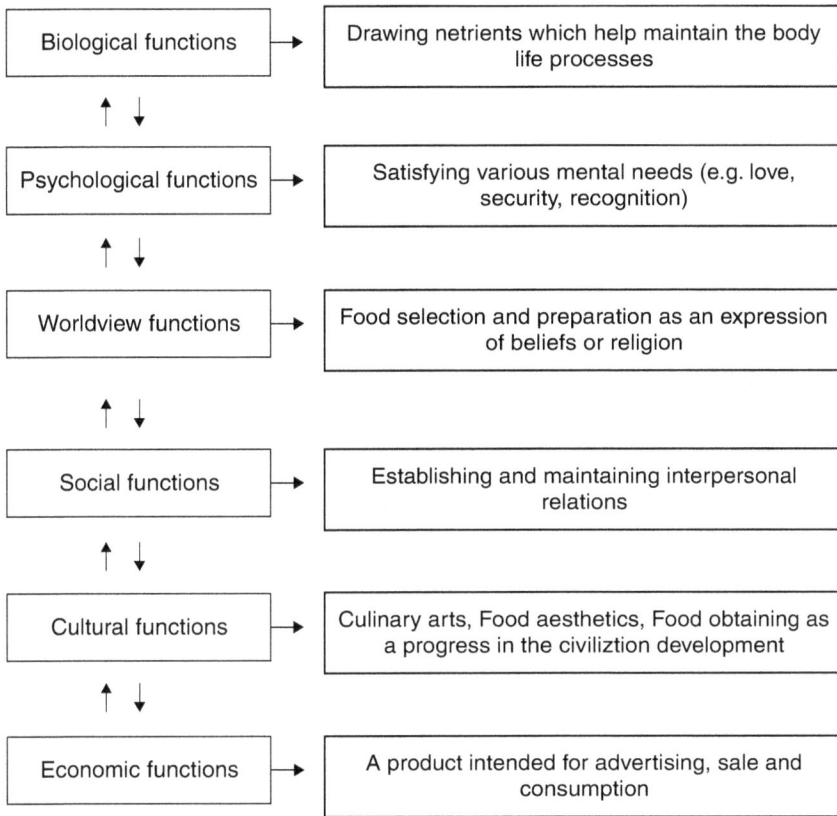

Figure 1.2 Functions of food (Niewiadomska et al., 2005; *Jedzenie. Uzależnienia: fakty i mity* [Food. Addictions: Facts and myths], p. 43. Wydawnictwo KUL).

deliberately limit their food intake because it is the only thing they can control (Niewiadomska et al., 2005). A person's cognitive beliefs about the nature and function of food and eating in the context of his importance for body image may be significantly influenced by family myths passed on through many generations, strongly rooted in family identity as well as significantly influencing the emerging habits and anti-health behaviors toward eating and the body.

Therefore, in the diagnosis of body image in eating disorders, it is important to include the basic indicators of the functions of eating in the patient's family in order to answer the following questions: (a) to what extent have myths and family messages about maladaptive patterns of behaviors toward food been internalized by the patient and (b) when do they become a regulator of an excessively restrictive/bulimic attitude toward food due to not accepting one's own body image.

Symbolic functions of food: diagnostic indicators

A preoccupation with food often performs symbolic functions, indicating the need to maintain a relationship or receive love or consolation from significant others. It can also express the pursuit of entertainment, pleasure, relaxation, or release internal tension. Often, verbal and nonverbal messages from significant others (especially from the mother, father, or other caregiver) reinforce the meaning of food as an expression of love and care and enhance the development of dependence. Regular messages such as "I'm doing it all for you," "I'm cooking this delicious food for you," or "I made this delicious dinner just for you," and so forth carry an implication that food is often a symbol and/or substitute for parental/maternal love. Love understood this way is not conducive to the process of separation and individuation in adolescence and early adulthood (Józefik, 2008; Józefik et al., 2010).

Eating can also be a sign of the emotional bond between a child and its parents. From its birth, the mother feeds and grooms the child in very close bodily contact, which strengthens their psychological bond and enhances the relationship between breastfeeding, emotional closeness, and the child's total dependence on the mother (Iniewicz et al., 2002; Józefik et al., 2002; Krueger, 2002a). Later in life, feeding may be associated with a specific type of emotional bond, often bearing the hallmarks of an emotional dependence that is too strong and does not allow for the proper course of separation and individuation during adolescence. Obviously, this is not conducive to directly expressing and experiencing the youthful rebellion so necessary at this stage of development. In such cases, a passive rebellion might emerge instead, hidden, for example, in the form of diseases or disorders. Eating can also be a sign of comforting. It is common in our culture to associate food with obtaining maternal comfort. For example, a teenager, and later an adult, learns to react in situations of stress and increased internal tension to by "longing for food" (overeating). The learned pattern of associating food with comfort is often the only available and relatively easy method of relieving emotional suffering. In this way, many emotional needs are vicariously satisfied (Czepczor & Brytek-Matera, 2017; Izydorczyk & Mazur, 2012). So-called myths about food are an especially important part of the patients' family relationships. The diverse content of these myths can stimulate many behaviors that the patients undertake toward their body and food. In family relationships, food can be an important source of unconscious compensation of mental (emotional) needs and behaviors that the individual is unable to meet or implement in a more adequate and mature way. In the course of family life and the relationships that develop there, feeding can become an important way of expressing love and care, especially between the child and the mother or other significant caregiver. Especially for adolescents, this pattern of treating food as a symbolic satisfaction of emotional needs of themselves or other people (e.g., feeding their fiancé) can transfer into adulthood.

Eating begins to function as a tension-reducing "comforter," but it can also be an expression of fear of responsibility and adulthood. Food is sometimes used by parents as an educational reinforcer – reward or punishment. Rewarding with food begins from early childhood and is a frequent way of enforcing the so-called desired behaviors (e.g., "When you clean the room, I will order a pizza/get you an ice cream," etc.). Punishment with food most often occurs in a refusal to eat a prepared meal. It is a punishment directed at the person preparing the meal. Refusal to eat a dish prepared by a loved one may be a way of communicating dissatisfaction regarding, for example, the marriage (Niewiadomska et al., 2005).

A refusal to eat (fasting) can be treated as a symbolic severing of relationships. Giving up certain meals (or completely depriving oneself of food) is sometimes a manifestation of self-punishment for certain behaviors or experienced emotions. In the family system, accepting or refusing meals may constitute a manifestation of control of one family member over the others, who then assumes the role of caring and protecting. Food can also be part of the art of seduction (i.e., showing interest and sympathy by inviting someone to a restaurant or preparing food especially for them). Food is also a substitute for a bond, and in some cases, can compensate for loneliness (Czepczor & Brytek-Matera, 2017).

In the psychological diagnosis of the functions of eating in satisfying emotional and social needs, it is also worth paying attention to the patient's fat phobia (fear of gaining weight). Popular culture promotes models of beauty with unrealistic proportions, which provokes the "fear of being fat" in media recipients (Cash & Pruzinsky, 2004; Izydorczyk et al., 2020). It is worth examining and differentiating (a) the fear of being fat as the need to be thin according to sociocultural standards (being attractive and accepted) from (b) severe fat phobia, which reflects a high level of discrepancy between the real and the ideal body image, typical for eating disorders. The phenomenon of "fat talk" developing in western culture may be an example of fat phobia and a focus on negative, downward comparisons of own body image with the cultural ideal – especially among adolescent girls and young adult women. Fat talk has been described by Nichter and Vuckovic (1994). Shannon and Mills (2015) define fat talk as a form of self-degradation during which individuals criticize their weight, dimensions, body shape, or physical condition, often also addressing the subject of their nutrition and physical activity. The negative assessment of the body by girls and young women is revealed by messages such as "I am very fat" or "My bottom looks fat in these pants" (Shannon & Mills, 2015). The research literature cites theories explaining the mechanisms underlying fat talk. Bem's (1967) theory of self-perception (as opposed to the theory of cognitive dissonance) assumes that when people create their self-image, they use the same techniques that they do to learn about the attitudes of others. These techniques are based on inference, which, in turn, is based on observation (Bem, 1967; Shannon & Mills, 2015). Thus, on the basis of (observable) behaviors, people draw conclusions about others' as well as their own internal (un-observable) states. In this sense, when expressing criticism about their own appearance, a person may conclude that he feel dissatisfied with his ap-pearance, even in a situation where his body-related emotions were not originally negative. Frequent repetition of fat talk dialogs may make in-dividuals start to perceive themselves as physically unattractive and others as attractive, regardless of their actual own appearance and conformity with the cultural standards of beauty (Shannon & Mills, 2015). Fat talk is also explained by the aforementioned theory of body objectification. This is because the vast majority of such dialogs are conducted by women (Payne et al., 2010). In this context, fat talk is a behavioral manifestation of body-related emotions (fear, shame) which result from the belief that one's bodily appearance is not adapted to cultural norms and beauty standards. Engaging in fat talk is intended to highlight the awareness of one's own imperfection, alleviate potential criticism, and reduce fear and shame (Shannon & Mills, 2015). Fat talk is most often observed among adolescent girls (Britton et al., 2006) and women in young adulthood (Martz et al., 2009) in western countries (Payne et al., 2010). It is characterized by dis-satisfaction with one's body image, the desire to lose weight despite having a statistically average or below-average BMI, glorification of slim figures, and a tendency toward social comparisons (Corning & Gondoli, 2012; Engel & Salk, 2014). It is possible that such conversations affect the development of body image distortions, ultimately leading to dysmorphophobic disorders (Shannon & Mills, 2015). In individuals with a tendency toward dietary restrictions, it may increase the risk of eating disorders (Compeau & Ambwani, 2013).

Intense fat phobia is an important psychological symptom of eating dis-orders (Garner, 2004). Patients with anorexia or bulimia are afraid of gaining weight and see their body in a distorted way, "feeling fat" even when their BMI indicates a state of exhaustion. Sometimes, fat phobia reaches the intensity characteristic of phobic disorders and leads to extreme physical exhaustion. In other cases, it can be less severe, but fat phobia is always a potential risk factor of anorexia or bulimia. Fat phobia masks other im-portant internal conflicts regarding self-esteem, self-efficacy, and a sense of security and agency in life. Conflicts related to separation and individuation are most often described as the most primary and the oldest, based parti-cularly strongly on childhood emotional deficits, which create significant body image distortions. In psychoanalytical theories, the metapsychology of fat phobia is related to unresolved internal conflicts that result from fixa-tions at the developmental stage in which there is an ambivalent relationship with the mother, excessive maternal and/or paternal control, excessive focus on issues and behaviors related to eating, and where food serves a symbolic satisfaction of the need for love and safety (Józefik, 2008). Often, mothers of daughters with anorexia also have intense fears of being fat and exercise control over their children through food and eating. Fat phobia and the mechanisms of anorexia are further influenced by others in the patient's environment. In a phobic refusal to eat, patients with anorexia can starve themselves to death, while patients with a traditional phobic disorder does not drive themselves to such self-destruction.

In families where an anorexic model of functioning develops, the parents' fear of being fat causes a continuum of displacement and projection of conflicts over food from an early age. Over time, this process profoundly distorts the child's perception of food and eating. When female patients with anorexia begin to achieve age- and gender-appropriate BMI, they begin to menstruate, and a complex, disturbed body image makes itself felt. It manifests itself in a particularly intense fear of being fat. We can hypothesize that the return of menstruation also marks the return of the patients' femininity and sexuality, from which they perhaps unconsciously tried to "escape" into a child's body and figure. The psychological basis of eating disorders is often considered to involve unresolved issues of separation and individuation (fear of autonomy, assuming the adult social role). Impulse control and fat phobia usually manifest differently in patients with the restricting subtype of anorexia than in those with the binging/purging subtype. In the latter group, inadequate impulse control periodically leads to binge eating, vomiting, substance use, and acting out. In many cases, internal conflicts are transferred onto the body and food (McDougall, 2014). Blocking sexual feelings and fantasies in girls predisposes them to greater conflict repression in the sphere of sexuality. Fat phobia hides the fear of regression in women. Patients with anorexia usually deny the needs related to emotional intimacy and properly manifested (i.e., without fear) dependence in relationships (Izydorczyk, 2015; Krueger, 2002b).

In sum, the psychological diagnosis of body image should consider the developmental function of food in satisfying the social and emotional needs of patients with eating disorders. Usually, satisfying a child's emotional needs through food is associated with emotional conflicts and centers around body image. Emotional conflicts most often concern the specificity of separation and individuation, from childhood through adolescence to adulthood. Difficulties in the proper course of separation and individuation most often appear in adolescence and often require an in-depth diagnosis of family and sociocultural predictors of anorexic and/or bulimic behaviors.

References

American Psychiatric Association. (2013). *Diagnostic and statistical manual of mental disorders* (5th ed.). 10.1176/appi.books.9780890425596

Bem, D. J. (1967). Self-perception: An alternative interpretation of cognitive dissonance phenomena. *Psychological Review, 74*(3), 183–200. 10.1037/h0024835

Britton, L. E., Martz, D. M., Bazzini, D. G., Curtin, L. A., & LeaShomb, A. (2006). Fat talk and self-presentation of body image: Is there a social norm for women to self- degrade? *Body Image, 3*(3), 247–254. 10.1016/j.bodyim.2006.05.006

Cash, T. F. (2004). Body image: Past, present, and future. *Body Image, 1*(1), 1–5. 10.1016/S1740-1445(03)00011-1

Cash, T. F. (2012). Cognitive-behavioral perspectives on body image. In T. F. Cash (Ed.), *Encyclopedia of body image and human appearance* (pp. 334–342). Academic Press.

Cash, T. F., & Pruzinsky T. (Eds.). (2004). *Body image. A handbook of theory, research, and clinical practice* (pp. 235–242). The Guilford Press.

Cash, T. F., & Smolak, L. (2011). Understanding body images: Historical and contemporary perspectives. In T. F. Cash, & L. Smolak (Eds.), *Body image: A handbook of science, practice, and prevention* (pp. 3–11). The Guilford Press.

Clarkin, J. F., Fonagy, P., & Gabbard, G. (2013). *Psychoterapia psychodynamiczna zaburzeń osobowości* [Psychodynamic psychotherapy of personality disorders]. Wydawnictwo Uniwersytetu Jagiellońskiego.

Compeau, A. & Ambwani, S. (2013). The effects of fat talk on body dissatisfaction and eating behavior: The moderating role of dietary restraint. *Body Image, 10*(4), 451–461. 10.1016/j.bodyim.2013.04.006

Corning, A. F., & Gondoli, D. M. (2012). Who is most likely to fat talk? A social comparison perspective. *Body Image, 9*(4), 528–531. 10.1016/j.bodyim.2012.05.004

Czepczor, K., & Brytek-Matera, A. (2017). *Jedzenie pod wpływem emocji* [Emotional eating]. Difin.

Domaradzki, J. (2013). O definicjach zdrowia i choroby [On the definitions of health and disease]. *Folia Medica Lodziensia, 40*(1), 5–29.

Encyklopedia PWN (2018). Eating, In *Encyklopedia PWN* (2018). Wydawnictwo Naukowe.

Engel, R., & Salk, R. H. (2014). The demographics of fat talk in adult women: Age, body size, and ethnicity. *Journal of Health Psychology, 21*(8), 1655–1664. 10.1177/1359105314560918

Fredrickson, B. L., & Roberts T. A. (1997). Objectification theory. Toward understanding women's lived experiences and mental health risks. *Psychology of Women Quarterly, 21*(2), 173–206. 10.1111/j.1471-6402.1997.tb00108.x

Gabbard, G. (2015). *Psychiatria psychodynamiczna w praktyce klinicznej* [Psychodynamic psychiatry in clinical practice]. Wydawnictwo Naukowe Uniwersytetu Jagiellońskiego.

Garner, D. M. (2004). *EDI-3. Eating Disorders Inventory. Professional Manual.* Psychological Assessment Resources, Inc.

Glickauf-Hughes Ch., & Wells M. (1997). *Object relations psychotherapy. An individual and integreative approach to diagnosis and treatment.* Jason Aronson, Inc.

Higgins, E. T. (1987). Self-discrepancy: A theory relating self and affect. *Psychological Review, 94*(3), 319–340.

Iniewicz, G., Józefik, B., Namysłowska, I., & Ulasińska, R. (2002). Obraz relacji rodzinnych w oczach pacjentek chorujących na anoreksję psychiczną - częśc II [The subjective picture of family relations in female anorexia patients – Part II]. *Psychiatria Polska, 1*, 65–81.

Izydorczyk, B. (2010). Psychoterapia oparta na teorii relacji z obiektem i psychodramie: integracyjne podejście w leczeniu zaburzeń odżywiania. [Object relations- and psychodrama-based psychotherapy: An integrative approach to the treatment of eating disorders]. *Psychiatria Polska, 44*(5), 677–691.

Izydorczyk, B. (2011). A psychological profile of the bodily self characteristics in women suffering from bulimia nervosa. In P. Hay (Ed.), *New insights into the prevention and treatment of bulimia nervosa* (pp. 147–167). Intech Open Access Publisher.

Izydorczyk, B. (2013a). A psychological diagnosis of the structure of the body self in a group. *Archives of Psychiatry and Psychotherapy, 2*, 21–306.

Izydorczyk, B. (2013b). Selected psychological traits and body image characteristics in females suffering from binge eating disorder. *Archives of Psychiatry and Psychotherapy, 15*(1), 19–33.

Izydorczyk, B. (2015). *Postawy i zachowania wobec własnego ciała w zaburzeniach odżywiania* [Attitudes and behaviors towards the body in eating disorders]. PWN.

Izydorczyk B. (2017a). Trauma in relation to psychological characteristics in women with eating disorders. *Current Issues in Personality Psychology, 5*(4), 244–259. 10.5114/cipp.2017.67047

Izydorczyk, B. (2017b). Psychoterapia zaburzeń obrazu ciała w anoreksji i bulimii psychicznej: podejście integracyjne (zastosowanie terapii psychodynamicznej i technik psychodramy) [Psychotherapy of body image distortions in anorexia and bulimia: An integrative approach (using elements of psychodynamic psychotherapy and psychodrama techniques)]. *Psychoterapia, 1*(180), 5–22.

Izydorczyk, B., & Mazur, K. (2012). Characteristics of aggressive behaviour in females suffering from psychogenic binge eating disorder (analysis of the author's own research). *Archives of Psychiatry and Psychotherapy, 14*(3), 15–24.

Izydorczyk, B., & Sitnik-Warchulska, K. (2018). Sociocultural appearance standards and risk factors for eating disorders in adolescents and women of various ages. *Frontiers in Psychology, 9*(429), 1–21. 10.3389/fpsyg.2018.00429

Izydorczyk, B., Sitnik-Warchulska, K., Lizińczyk, S., & Lipowska, M. (2020). Socio-cultural standards promoted by the mass media as predictors of restrictive and bulimic behavior. *Frontiers in Psychiatry, 11*(506), 1–14. 10.3389/fpsyt.2020. 00506

Józefik, B. (2008). Koncepcja przywiązania a zaburzenia odżywiania – teoria i empiria [Attachment and eating disorders – theory and empirical results]. *Psychiatria Polska, 42*(2), 157–166.

Józefik, B. (2014). *Kultura, ciało, (nie)jedzenie* [Culture, body, (not)eating]. Wydawnictwo Uniwersytetu Jagiellońskiego.

Józefik, B., Iniewicz, G., Namysłowska, I., & Ulasińska, R. (2002). Obraz relacji rodzinnych w oczach pacjentek chorujących na anoreksję psychiczną – część I [The subjective picture of family relations in female anorexia patients – Part I]. *Psychiatria Polska, 36*(1), 51–64.

Józefik, B., Iniewicz, G., & Ulasińska, R. (2010). Wzory przywiązania, samoocena i płeć psychologiczna w anoreksji i bulimii psychicznej [Attachment patterns, self-esteem, and psychological gender in anorexia and bulimia]. *Psychiatria Polska, 44*(5), 665–676.

Krueger, D. W. (2002a). Psychodynamic perspective on body image. In T. F. Cash, & T. Pruzinsky (Eds.), *Body image. A handbook of theory, research, and clinical practice* (pp. 30–37). The Guilford Press.

Krueger, D. W. (2002b). *Integrating body self and psychological self. Creating a new story in psychoanalysis and psychotherapy.* Bruner-Routledge.

Krystal, H. (2000). *Trauma und Affekte – Posttraumtische Folgeerscheinungen und ihre Konsequenzen für die psychoanalytische Behandlungstechnik.* [Paper presentation]. Contemporary sychoanalysis. Frankfurt, Germany.

Lemma, A. (2014). *Pod skórą psychoanalityczne studium modyfikacji ciała* [Under the skin. A psychoanalytic study of body modification]. Imago.

Lemma, A. (2016). *Ciało w umyśle. Rozważania o ciele w psychoanalizie i w programach telewizyjnych* [Body in the mind. Reflections on the body in psychoanalysis and in television programs]. Oficyna Ingenium.

Madowitz, J., Matheson, B. E., & Liang, J. (2015). The relationship between eating disorders and sexual trauma. *Eating and Weight Disorders, 20,* 281–293. 10.1007/s40519-015-0195-y

Martz, D. M., Petroff, A. B., Curtin, L. A., & Bazzini, D. G. (2009). Gender differences in fat talk among American adults: Results from the psychology of size survey. *Sex Roles, 61,* 34–41. 10.1007/s11199-009-9587-7

McDougall, J. (2014). *Teatr ciała. Psychoanalityczne podejście do chorób psychosomatycznych* [Theatre of the body: A psychoanalytic approach to psychosomatic illness]. Oficyna Ingenium.

McWilliams, N. (2014). *Diagnoza psychoanalityczna* [Psychoanalytic diagnosis]. Gdańskie Wydawnictwo Psychologiczne.

Mikołajczyk, E., & Samochowiec, J. (2004a). Cechy psychologiczne pacjentek z zaburzeniami odżywiania w porównaniu ze studentkami wyższych szkół medycznych badanych kwestionariuszem EDI [Personality characteristics of female patients with eating disorders compared to female students of medical schools measured by the EDI questionnaire]. *Psychiatria Polska, 38,* 170–171.

Mikołajczyk, E., & Samochowiec, J. (2004b). Cechy osobowości u pacjentek z zaburzeniami odżywiania [Personality characterisitcs of female patients with eating disorders]. *Psychiatria, 1*(2), 91–95.

Nichter, M., & Vuckovic, N. (1994). Fat talk: Body image among adolescent girls. In N. Sault (Ed.), *Many mirrors: Body image and social relations* (pp. 109–131). Rutgers University Press.

Niewiadomska, I., Kulik, A., & Hajduk, A. (2005). *Jedzenie. Uzależnienia: fakty i mity.* [Eating. Addictions: Facts and myths]. Wydawnictwo Gaudium.

Payne, L. O., Martz, D., Nezami, B. T., & Farrow, C. V. (2010). Gender comparisons of fat talk in the United Kingdom and the United States. *Sex Roles, 65*(7), 557–565. 10.1007/s11199-010-9881-4

Rodgers, R. F., Slater, A., & Gordon, Ch. S. (2020). Biopsychosocial model of social media use and body image concerns, disordered eating, and muscle-building behaviors among adolescent girls and boys. *Journal of Youth and Adolescence, 49,* 399–409. 10.1007/s10964-019-01190-0

Sakson-Obada, O. (2008). Rozwój Ja cielesnego w kontekście wczesnej relacji z opiekunem [Development of the body Ego in the context of the early relationship with a caregiver]. *Roczniki Psychologiczne, 11,* 27–44.

Sakson-Obada, O. (2009a). *Pamięć ciała. Ja cielesne w relacji przywiązania i w traumie* [The body's memory. The body Self in attachment relationships and trauma]. Wydawnictwo Difin.

Sakson-Obada, O. (2009b). Trauma jako czynnik ryzyka dla zaburzeń Ja cielesnego [trauma as a risk factor for the disorders of the bodily ego]. *Przegląd Psychologiczny, 52,* 309–326.

Schier, K. (2010). *Piękne brzydactwo. Psychologiczna problematyka obrazu ciała i jego zaburzeń* [Ugly beauty. The psychology of body image and its disorders]. Wydawnictwo Naukowe Scholar.

Shannon, A., & Mills, J. S. (2015). Correlates, causes, and consequences of fat talk: A review. *Body Image*, *15*, 158–172. 10.1016/j.bodyim.2015.09.003

Skrzypska, N., & Suchańska, A. (2011). Uraz seksualny jako czynnik ryzyka zaburzeń doświadczania własnej cielesności [Sexual trauma as a risk factor of disorders in experiencing of one's own body]. *Seksuologia Polska*, *9*(2), 51–56.

Södersten, U., Brodin, M., Zandian, C. & Bergh (2019). Eating behavior and the evolutionary perspective on anorexia nervosa. *Frontiers in Neuroscience*, *13*:596. 10.3389/fnins.2019.00596

Terhoeven, V., Nikendei, Ch., Bärnighausen, T., Bountogo, M., Friederich, H. Ch., Ouermi, L., Sié, A., & Harling, G. (2020). Eating disorders, body image and media exposure among adolescent girls in rural Burkina Faso. *Tropical Medicine and International Health*, *25*(1), 132–142. 10.1111/tmi.13340

Thompson, J. K., & Smolak, L. (2001). *Body image, eating disorders, and obesity in youth: Assessment, prevention and treatment.* American Psychological Association.

Vartanian, L. E., Hayward, J.M., Smyth, S. J., Paxton, S., & Touyz, S. W. (2018). Risk and resiliency factors related to body dissatisfaction and disordered eating: The identity disruption model. *International Journal of Eating Disorders*, *51*(4), 322–330. 10.1002/eat.22835

Wertheim, E. H., Paxton, S. J., & Blaney, S. (2004). Risk factors for the development of body image disturbances. In J. K. Thompson (Ed.), *Handbook of eating disorders and obesity* (p. 463–494). John Wiley & Sons.

World Health Organization. (1993). *The ICD-10 classification of mental and behavioural disorders.* World Health Organization.

World Health Organization. (2018). *International classification of diseases for mortality and morbidity statistics*(11th Revision). https://icd.who.int/browse11/l-m/en

2 Family and sociocultural predictors of body image development

The social environment is a significant source of numerous sociocultural and family messages concerning body image and attitudes toward food and eating. Beginning from childhood, through adolescence and young adulthood, peer and family messages are internalized as important sources of knowledge which impact the relationship between the attitudes related to food and eating and those related to the body. Thus, it is important to identify and highlight the important role of family myths and messages concerning body image and eating together with the patterns of emotional relationships (especially between children and parents) in shaping behaviors toward the body and eating. Chapter 2 also presents the of psychological profiles describing the specificity of the sociocultural indices of body image among young women and men is an important element in the psychological diagnosis of the risk of dysfunctions in experiencing one's own body, which might facilitate the development of anorexic readiness, bigorexia, or other anti-health eating behaviors.

Family and social myths and messages about food and body image

Apart from the above-mentioned select features of families of patients with eating disorders, their psychological diagnosis should also include their families' myths and messages about food and their role in the family system. Often the specificity of the family message is related to the body image myths held by the patient. The myths functioning in the family system may relate to many taboo topics, repeated statements, or proverbs (Niewiadomska et al., 2005). Family messages about food play an important role in influencing the understanding of its psychosocial functions. They are often an element of communication between family members and the patient. They constitute a unit of well-organized beliefs that the family members share and apply to each other. They are used to maintain the family *status quo* as well as – especially in times of crisis – its directions and patterns of change. A family myth can create a homeostatic mechanism. It is triggered when the tension between family members reaches a point where it (objectively or in

DOI: 10.4324/9781003251088-2

the family members' perception) threatens intrafamily relationships. It functions as an "inner image" to which all family members contribute and which they try to maintain. It describes the roles and responsibilities of individual family members in their mutual relations. A family myth performs the same function as an individual defense mechanism. It likewise plays an important role in interactions with the outside world. When the myth is shaken by various events and circumstances, the individuals' defense systems are also shaken (Ostoja-Zawadzka, 1999).

Family stories often include scripts and legends. Family scripts usually describe a detailed pattern of interaction, that is, a sequence of behaviors related to specific events (e.g., in connection with cooking, preparing family celebrations at home). It can be compared to the cognitive representation of family relationships that the patient transfers to the matrix of his own behaviors toward the body and food. On the other hand, family legends are select stories from family life, for example, about food, body image standards, and various related experiences propagated across generations. As they often take the form of moral parables, they dictate how family members should behave toward the body and food, both in their own lives and in relation to others. From the individual perspective, myths can be compared with cognitive schemas that determine thinking, perception, memory, and behavior. For patients with eating disorders, whose body image is inextricably linked with their approach to eating and their emotional experience of food, the importance of family messages in this area is clear. On the one hand, family myths often refer to identity and the psychosexual role, and on the other, they influence the expectations regarding the definition, method, and likelihood of achieving attractiveness (Józefik, 1999).

Food myths are passed down across generations not only through the family system, but also through mass media. Some myths propagated by media concern the perception of thinness and overweight. Research on obesity indicates that being overweight in adulthood is unhealthy. The ideal of female attractiveness has also changed, as thin women are usually described as beautiful (Niewiadomska et al., 2005). Among the myths and family messages about food, the following may appear:

- a chubby child is a healthy child;
- as long as the child has the correct weight, there is no need to worry about eating habits;
- the child is growing, so childhood overweight does not pose a health risk;
- losing weight is harmful to the child's health;
- every diet is healthy;
- every diet is more or less effective;
- the use of diets is safe for the psyche;
- the use of diuretics and laxatives allows to lose weight quickly;
- achieving the desired weight is the basis for happiness and self-confidence.

I am losing weight, so I change myself and my life for the better – being overweight is a sign of failure in life, and being thin is a sign of success – one has to be slim to be happy and attractive. Adolescents who cannot cope with the stress of everyday life often escape into so-called surrogate behaviors. When they cannot build and maintain peer relationships, they take the position of a scapegoat, someone who is always on the sidelines, with a poorer academic record. People may also feel alienated because of very good academic results, a high social position in the group (though associated only with school achievement), but a body weight exceeding the cultural norm (they are called chubby or fat). They begin, often unconsciously, to look for a strategy of coping with this situation. They experience difficult emotions such as anger, uncertainty, shame, and fear, and they must discharge them in a socially approved way. They begin to control their weight in an attempt to achieve a positive change in their life ("I will be thinner, I will be more attractive to others, they will like me, I will have friends, others will admire me"). *I can keep a perfect figure, although I cannot be perfect in everything–* a young person in an emotionally difficult situation (crisis of adolescence, family or marital conflicts, related, for example to the breakdown of the emotional bond between the partners, divorce, the father's growing conflict relationship, excessive or insufficient parental control) wants to prove that he is important, he can meet the expectations he faces, and he is perfect. The so-called empty nest syndrome (the parents' lack of readiness to accept their adolescent child's separation, thus sending them "stay at home" signals) may also facilitate internal conflict in the adolescent manifested in the sphere of the body and body image. Weight control and maintaining a figure which, according to the dominant social narrative, guarantees success in the peer group, are supposed to help the adolescent feel appreciated and perfect (competent). This is often the only way of compensating for the experienced internal conflicts and the feeling of a lack of influence in life. Low self-esteem and a lack of agency in the unacceptable family situation may lead to a "defensive escape" into perfectionism, excessive weight control, and a resulting recognition of one's perfection ("in other areas of my life, perfection is impossible"). The search for a sense of value and acceptance as well as success in losing weight results from conflicting expectations for adolescent children. On the one hand, adults communicate to their female children the need for independence and professional success, and, on the other hand, the need to assume the traditional female role of the subservient caregiver. Other, frequent parental messages include "you have the right not to rush long-term relationships, you have time for that, take care of your needs, do not 'tie the knot' too fast." At the same time, the social environment endorses such messages as: "a lonely girl without friends or relationships with the opposite sex has something wrong with her." *After all, I can live up to social demands despite everything. I must do this.* Often endorsed by the social environment, the prescriptions regarding the maintenance of a thin body shape function in an equally conflicting relationship: "you must stay

thin in a world of choice and excess." In this context of social communication, another prescriptive myth develops: "take care of your interests
and needs" but also "satisfy, above all, the needs of others, otherwise you
will be selfish." "You have to be feminine, but also, being the way you are is
not okay, you have to constantly correct and change your body." Becoming
an adult woman is not pleasant or easy. An unconscious desire not to grow
up might develop. Anorexia plays an important role in this desire. As a
result of a restrictive diet, the body does not develop, and it resembles the
figure of a teenage girl dependent on her parents. Faced with such contradictory, often implicit expectations, young women can feel that every choice
they make is wrong. On the other hand, the goal of becoming thin seems
clear and achievable. "If I cannot be everything they want me to be, I can at
least look as perfect as if I achieved it all." *Anorexia nervosa* literally means
"lack of appetite" for psychological reasons. However, this name does not
reflect the true nature of this disorder, and even contradicts it. The anorexic
person has a great need for food, and this is his chief concern. Giving in to
one's own needs causes panic, fear, and dread so great that it takes the form
of a food phobia, an obsession with not eating/eating. Instead of eating
food, the anorexic patients realize this need by fantasizing about eating or
feeding others. Sometimes, they succumb to this need by eating a large
amount of food in a short time (binging), and then purging in various ways.
Weight loss is experienced as a success, it becomes proof of competence,
strength, and endurance, while gaining weight becomes a failure, shame, and
loss of self-control. Therefore, patients with anorexia have no choice but to
deny that anything harmful is happening to them because, paradoxically, the
disorder may make them feel valuable. One could say that up to a certain
point, the patients experience more "benefits" (described above) than health
costs. In the face of losses, they sometimes remain uncritical. Only the
breakdown of social and family life, the loss of social position at school, or
the feeling that the disease takes up 90%–100% of thoughts and life activities, leaving no room for anything else, leads the patients to start treatment
and look for a different, nondestructive way to gain the feeling of being
complete, independent, and competent. Otherwise, the life of an anorexic
patient focuses on eating at the expense of every other sphere (relationships,
family, own interests, school, work), leading to mental deterioration (cognitive problems, depression, insomnia, suicidal thoughts), physical exhaustion, and, in extreme cases, death.

As can be seen, it appears that in these emotionally difficult situations,
food has a symbolic function for adolescents, being an expression of unmet
needs and a failure to cope with cultural pressures concerning beauty.

Attachment patterns and body image

As indicated by Bowlby's attachment theory (1988), Fonagy's mentalization
theory, and object relations theory (especially Mahler's separation–individuation

theory), the development of the experience of corporeality is influenced by patterns of early childhood attachment to their caregiver (Schier, 2020). The attachment pattern becomes an important factor explaining the so-called safe and unsafe (emotionally unstable) ways of establishing relations between the child's body and the caregiver's body. It determines the way of establishing social relations in adulthood (Bowlby, 2021). The trusting (secure) attachment pattern provides the basis for the development of the correct proportion of closeness (emotional as well as bodily) between the child and its caregiver (Schier, 2020). People who have experienced insecure relationship patterns in the course of their childhood development and their relationship with the caregiver may also develop a maladaptive (insecure) relationship with their own body. Schier (2020) introduced the term "loneliness of the body." It refers to the bodily experience of children and adolescents as a state of disruption of trust in the early childhood relationship with the caregiver. A child whose body was loved, accepted, and cared for will love, accept, and care for their body later in life (Kearney-Cooke, 2002; Patton et al., 2014; Schier, 2020).

The importance of the quality of the caregiver's touch in the relationship with the child for the shaping of the adult's body experience is indicated by Głowacka (2020), while the importance of physical closeness and bond for the development of body image in school children and adolescents is also emphasized in the latest Polish research by Schier (2020). The parents' body image beliefs held by the adolescent are a significant risk factor of eating disorders (Schier, 2020). Family determinants in the genesis, course, and treatment of eating disorders are widely researched and described in the literature (Cerniglia et al., 2017; Treasure & Todd, 2016). One of the most important aspects in this area is the relationship between children and parents, which is most often studied based on attachment theory (Balottin et al., 2017; Monteleone et al., 2019; Schier, 2020; Tasca, 2019; Tasca & Balfour, 2014; Tasca et al., 2009). A systematic review of 24 studies by Tetley et al. (2014) clearly shows that women diagnosed with eating disorders (as well as patients with other psychiatric diagnoses) are much more likely to report poorer quality of bond with their parents compared to those without a psychiatric diagnosis. The studies by Izydorczyk et al., conducted in 2018–2020 (in the course of preparing this book) on a population of 134 teenagers aged 12–19 years, verified, among other things, whether the perception of parental bond explains body image. To measure the perception of parental bond, Izydorczyk et al. (in press) used the *Parental Bonding Instrument* (PBI) questionnaire developed by Parker et al. (1979; Parker, 1998), translated by Agnieszka Popiel and Monika Sitarzsee (see Popiel & Pragłowska, 2006). The *Multidimensional Body-Self Relations Questionnaire* (MBSRQ) by Thomas F. Cash (Brytek-Matera & Rogoza, 2015; Cash & Grasso, 2005; Cash & Pruzinsky, 2004) was used to diagnose body image. On the other hand, to measure sociocultural attitudes toward appearance, the authors used the Polish adaptation of *The Sociocultural Attitudes*

Towards Appearance Questionnaire (SATAQ 3) by Thompson and Gray (1995) in polish adaptation (see Izydorczyk & Lizińczyk, 2020). Results of a regression analysis (see Izydorczyk et al., in press) indicated that the perception of the parental bond (especially the quality of maternal care) and body image are significant risk factors of eating disorders. The risk factors in the area of body image in relation to various aspects of eating disorders were the satisfaction with body appearance, care for appearance, and care for physical fitness. The higher the satisfaction with body appearance, the lower the tendency to control weight and engage in restrictive and bulimic behaviors. Many studies to date also indicate that insecure attachment patterns in relationships with caregivers are risk factors of eating disorders (Gander et al., 2015; Salcuni et al., 2017; Tetley et al., 2014). Moreover, as indicated by Bowlby and Fonagy, insecure attachment styles negatively influence the development of cognitive-affective structures related to interpersonal relationships and the experience of specific emotions (Bowlby, 1988; Bowlby & Ainsworth, 1965; Fonagy et al., 2007; Fonagy et al., 2013, 2015). Research by Józefik et al. (2010) highlighted the experience of particularly difficult maternal relationships in patients with eating disorders. The importance of the quality of the relationship with the caregiver and the relationship to food and eating is also indicated by the growing role of fathers in raising children compared to previous periods. The role of the father is extremely important in shaping adolescents' identity and self-esteem (Enten & Golan, 2009). In most of the studies using the PBI, maternal and paternal overprotection was a risk factor of eating disorders, particularly in patients with binge eating disorder and general eating problems (Tetley et al., 2014).

Psychological and especially psychoanalytical theories point to a link between the attachment pattern developed in childhood and the dominant patterns of establishing emotional relationships in adulthood (Bowlby, 1988; Bowlby & Ainsworth, 1965; Glickauf-Hughes & Wells, 1997). Bowlby's attachment theory concerns the innate tendency to form strong bonds with caregivers. Attachment describes a specific child–caregiver relationship, usually from the child's perspective. The parents' perspective is reflected in the dimension of parental care (Bowlby, 1988; Bowlby & Ainsworth, 1965). Repeated parent–child interactions shape the so-called internal working models (mental structures) that influence the child's further development, their perception of themselves and the world, the course of their socialization, and the formation of self-esteem and agency (Bowlby, 1988). As psychosomatic theories and contemporary psychoanalytical theories concerning the development of the body Self indicate, the parents' emotional response patterns influence the child's development of the basic personality structure, which includes the body Self, the basis for the mental Self. According to Krueger (2002a, 2002b), the following basic features of the parent–child relationship in early childhood indicate predispositions toward developing body image distortions in adulthood:

1. Intrusiveness and overstimulation by the caregiver (an attempt to regulate emotions, reduce tension, and restore control over the body).
2. Emotional inaccessibility and lack of empathy (the child cannot become a point of reference for themselves. Later, the basic experiences of bodily boundaries are created through impulsive behaviors or substance use. Internal body awareness is also increased through such behaviors as fasting, binge eating, purging, and compulsive physical exercise).
3. The inconsistency and selectivity of responding to the child's needs (the parents focus on the child's physical needs and pain, ignoring kinesthetic or emotional stimuli) allow the child to learn that in order to gain the parents' interest and acceptance, he should organize his experiences around the physical matters related to pain and illness. In such a situation, emotions never desomatize – they are felt only at the level of their physical component, and the pattern of experiencing the body and mental Self also develops through the prism of pain and illness (psychosomatic disorders, including eating disorders).

Krueger (2002a, 2002b) also draws attention to the influence of the caregiver–child relationship on body image disorders. There are three types of relational patterns. The first is parental overprotection, control, and intrusiveness. Such upbringing limits the child's agency and deprives him of the chance to develop autonomy. It can also inhibit of development and facilitate disorders of experiencing oneself and one's body, including anorexia. The body is then perceived as immature, asexual, and small. In stressful situations, individuals with such patterns of attachment might employ the defense mechanism of regression, self-harm, or engage in physical self-stimulation in order to reduce tension, regulate emotions, and restore the lost sense of control over the body.

Another relational pattern is empathic unavailability. The lack of a caring parent that would reflect the child's inner states leads to the child's inability to find support within himself. The caregiver's care and touch define the boundaries of the child's body, teaching him how to recognize internal signals. People who have not experienced such a relationship in early childhood see their bodies as too large and shapeless in adulthood. Their body image changes frequently throughout the day depending on their mood. They might engage in substance use and compulsive behaviors to acquire basic experiences related to bodily boundaries. These include damaging the skin surface or compulsive sex or masturbation. However, to increase internal bodily awareness, such patients often fast, binge or overeat, purge, and engage in compulsive exercise (Krueger, 2002a, 2002b).

The third type of parent–child relational pattern is selectivity and inconsistency. Difficulties in the development of symbolization arise when the caregiver selectively focuses on the child's physical needs and ailments, ignoring emotional needs. The pattern of experiencing the body Self through physical illness may cause a susceptibility to psychosomatic disorders. The child learns that in order to gain interest, he must organize his experiences around pain (Krueger, 2002a, 2002b). Care for and protection of the body are inseparable from the body Self. Taking care of one's own body is the result of a specific emotional relationship with it as well as the ability to properly receive and interpret bodily signals (Sakson-Obada, 2009a, 2009b).

Apart from Bowlby's (1988) attachment theory, the importance of the attachment pattern for the formation of personality is emphasized by mentalization theory (Fonagy et al., 2007). It posits that the ability to become aware of own and other people's mental states develops on the basis of early childhood relationships with significant others. Mental states become a subject of reflection, prompting the perception of other peoples' behavior as predictable and significant. This reflexivity is termed "autobiographical competence." Importantly, it enables the distinction between internal and external states, emotional regulation, impulse control, and the experience of oneself and the structure of one's Self (Fonagy et al., 2007, 2013). The pattern of the child's relationship with the caregiver is shaped by the caregiver's ability to recognize and verbalize messages sent by the child through the body. Bowlby (1988) suggests that the fine-tuning between the caregiver and the child is the basis of psychological bonding. It enables communication on a higher, verbal and symbolic level, giving the foundations for the differentiation of the body and mental Self (Krueger, 2002a, 2002b; Józefik, 2014; Schier, 2010).

In sum, attachment patterns are related to the development of body image and experience (Krueger, 2002a, 2002b). They also change later in life under the influence of individual social experiences, but their basis is formed in the relationship with caregivers in the first years of life (Krueger, 2002a, 2002b; Schier, 2010).

Diagnosis of the relationship pattern in families of patients with eating disorders

Denial of the need for emotional closeness and dependence is often determined by parental conflicts focused on weight, food, and expressions of aggression and other emotional states by the patient with eating disorders (Iniewicz et al. 2002; Józefik et al., 2002). The pattern of parental emotional responsiveness often includes compulsiveness, moralizing, and perfectionism. The important diagnostic indicator characteristics of specific types of families of patients with eating disorders are:

- overprotective families characterized by a high level of anxiety and a low degree of independence;
- "tight-knit" families, in which individual roles are incorrectly defined and implemented (disturbed family structure: dominant mother, weak husband/father), individual aspirations are suppressed, and subordination is expected;

- rigid families, in which there is a strong attachment to maintaining the unchanging *status quo* (defense mechanism) through avoidance, masking, denial, and concealing of significant conflicts;
- isolated families, hermetically closed off from the world (family members protect each other);
- families dominated by the parents' desire to become emotionally dependent on each other, and especially on their adolescent children (which results in limiting their autonomy and independence), where the children learn to suppress their own desires and needs;
- families in which addictions often occur in one of the parents, most often as a family secret (taboo topic);
- families with so-called "emotional selection": one child "belongs" to one parent, the other to the other (so-called division of children, such as: father's daughter, mother's son);
- families where there is excessive parental fear of obesity, dietary concerns, and perfectionism (excessive focus on children's good behavior and social conformism), and impulsivity.

Multigenerational family messages based on loyalty may be related to unfinished mourning associated with resignation, impulse control, strict demands, achievements, and a sense of justice (Józefik, 1999; Józefik et al., 2002). Among the significant patterns in the families of patients with eating disorders, the following are particularly important:

- disturbed boundaries in the family structure, where parents create a specific circle that separates them from other people, revealing difficulties in building interpersonal relationships, resolving conflicts, and reaching compromise;
- emotional dependence on the parents – especially by adolescent children (limiting their autonomy; love is understood as overprotection);
- meeting parents' expectations;
- suppressing one's own needs and desires (a compulsion combined with competing to show who is more devoted to other people);
- the principle of loyalty with caregivers – noncompliance with typical family behaviors causes guilt (Brytek-Matera, 2008).

Body image in mothers and daughters (comparative analysis)

The literature emphasizes the role of self-esteem in shaping body dissatisfaction (Wertheim et al., 2004). Body weight, thinness, and shape become the standards for self-worth (Garner, 2004). The influence of internalized family norms and the emotional bond with the parents on body image is indicated by contemporary cognitive (Cash, 2004; 2012) and psychoanalytical theories (Krueger, 2002a, 2002b). Domene et al. (2011) showed that, compared to mother–son relationships, mother–daughter relationships during the process of entering adulthood are characterized by fewer conflicts, more shared activities, and more open conversations, which may shape similarities. The influence of messages from the same-sex parent on body image in adolescents seems to also be confirmed by Izydorczyk (2010), who examined a group of young women with anorexia and their mothers. Many other studies published since 2000 also highlight the influence of social norms and messages on body image (Kearney-Cooke, 2002; Tantleff-Dunn & Gokee, 2002; Wertheim et al., 2004). Izydorczyk and Sitnik-Warchulska (2018) studied a population of mothers and their daughters and found that they similarly experienced a conflict between their real and ideal body image. The sample in the study consisted of 51 pairs of mothers (M = 55.5, SD = 3.39; BMI = 24.1, SD = 4.99) and daughters (M = 23, SD = 3.31; BMI = 24.94, SD = 3.39). The variable of social competence was defined as the personal efficacy in coping with significant social situations, such as intimate contacts (emotional and physical satisfaction with sexual intercourse), social exposure (voicing one's opinions), and assertiveness (i.e., the ability to set boundaries). Body esteem was defined as a construct comprising the discrepancy between the real and the ideal body image, self-assessed sexual attractiveness, physical fitness, and tendency toward weight control, both among the mothers and the daughters. Body esteem was measured with the Contour Drawing Rating Scale (Thompson & Gray, 1995) and the Body Esteem Scale (Franzoni & Shields, 1984) in a Polish adaptation by Lipowska and Lipowski (2013). Social competence was measured with the Social Competence Questionnaire (*Kwestionariusz Kompetencji Społecznych, KKS*) by Matczak (2007). Cronbach's α ranged between 0.74 and 0.94. The results showed no statistically significant differences between the mothers and their daughters regarding the discrepancy between the real and the ideal body image as well as between the real and the ought (socially mandated) body image. The mothers and their daughters in the sample experienced a similar intensity of conflict between their appraisals of their body image and their beliefs about how their bodies should look like.

The results of Izydorczyk and Sitnik-Warchulska (2018) also confirmed that the better the mothers' physical condition and the higher their discrepancy between their real and the ideal body image, the greater their general social competences. On the other hand, the higher the daughters' general self-esteem and the greater their discrepancy between their real and ideal body image, the higher their social competences. The empirically proven similarity of mothers' and daughters' beliefs about the socially expected body image as well as the similarity in their appraisals of their real body image may be related to biological and psychosocial processes (i.e., upbringing, modeling, internalization, pattern transmission). Additionally, body esteem, especially the discrepancy between the ideal and real body image, is an important predictor of social competences, as shown by Strauman and Higgins (1988) and Moretti and Higgins (1990, 1999).

The predictive significance of the discrepancy in social competences was indicated by Johns and Peters (2012). They emphasized that the discrepancy between the appraisal of the real body image (how the person perceives his body) and the assessment of the ought body image (how the body should look) reinforces the fear of establishing social relationships. Similar conclusions on the relationship between social competences and behaviors and attitudes toward food appear in Canadian research (O'Connor, 2000).

Uzunian and de Souza Vitalle (2015) reviewed 63 articles published between 2007 and 2013 which included American, Brazilian, and British samples, among others. They showed a relationship between adolescents' social competences and eating disorders: higher social competences are a protective factor against eating disorders in adolescents. On the other hand, Sepúlveda et al. (2020) studied a sample of 239 families and showed a relationship between loss of control over eating in children and dysfunctions in the family environment. The study measured family emotional expression, family adaptation and coherence levels, depression and anxiety symptoms in the children, self-esteem, and attitudes toward eating. Their results showed that overweight children had lower body esteem and showed higher stress and emotional engagement than did children with normal body mass index (BMI). Depression, anxiety, and disordered attitudes toward eating were partial mediators in the relationship between the expressed emotions and loss of control over eating.

Arroyo and Segrin (2013) studied young women and showed a relationship between family interactions and disordered attitudes toward eating, with a mediating role of social competences and psychological distress. The results showed that patterns of family interactions and family expressed emotions were related to low social competences, which led to psychological distress and the development of eating disorders.

In sum, a review of the literature shows a significant influence of social competences and family interactions on the development of pathological eating behaviors. Thus, the diagnosis and psychological therapy of patients with low body esteem and eating disorders should consider the specific emotional changes taking place in such patients' families.

Body dissatisfaction and emotional changes in the families of patients with eating disorders

As body dissatisfaction increases, along with other symptoms of eating disorders, the emotional states in the patients' immediate family environment (especially among parents and caregivers) also change. Family members experience various difficult emotional changes and go through challenging phases in the process of accepting a situation in which they unwillingly found themselves. The first phase in the development of eating disorders and growing body dissatisfaction as well as fat phobia centers around denial. The denial stage often masks the patient's fear and anxiety about the persistently incorrect body weight and body dissatisfaction. During this stage, the parent (guardian, partner) often experiences anxiety due to realizing the importance of the problem on the one hand (feeling responsible for the patient's disorder), and on the other hand, parent reacts defensively by "masking" it through behaviors that minimize or even neglect its importance. Common statements include "she is hysterical, she is stubborn, she is immature, she wants to prove something, it will pass when she gets older, everyone is on a diet at this age" and so forth. The overheard, although often incomplete knowledge of eating disorders often deepens the caregiver's guilt. As the symptoms of eating disorders develop, the second stage occurs, characterized by anger. The symptoms intensify. Restrictive fasting, slimming, fat phobia, induced vomiting (often hidden in bags), accumulation of hidden food, stealing money to buy food (to binge on and purge later), physical and/or verbal aggression, emotional hyperactivity, and irritability appear. Simultaneously, emotional terror in the parents and/or partners increases, leading to such questions as "why does he do it? why can't he stop?" Further claims follow, such as: "if he wanted, he would stop, if he loved me, he would stop hurting me, he is ruining his life," and so forth. Another stage that may appear in the relationship between a patient with an eating disorder and his immediate family members is the negotiation stage. It includes the parents or caregivers offering rewards to the patient for changing his behavior (e.g., "if you start to eat and gain weight, you will get....," "I will do whatever you ask for"), or making ultimatums ("if you do not stop doing it, you will not get pocket money, I will not pay for your school," etc.). When a parent or partner is unable to make the patient change his behaviors (body dissatisfaction, fat phobia, binging, and purging), he often experiences a deep sadness, guilt, and helplessness. Advanced stages of eating disorders and progress through the above stages might lead to acceptance of the disorder in the family. Parents, partners, or caregivers who do everything they can to help the patient must recognize and accept the fact that the ultimate responsibility rests with the patient themselves.

Psychological support for the family should emphasize the need for dialog with the patient. The following rules might be useful to share with the patient's parents/partner.

1. Decide who is the best person to talk to about body dissatisfaction and restrictive and/or compulsive eating behaviors (most often the mother). Discussions of those behaviors should be initiated and maintained by one person, otherwise the patient may become convinced that "everyone conspires against them" and have formed a coalition. This is not conducive to treatment, especially for adolescents, who are especially sensitive to external pressure and usually react with opposition.
2. Choose a time to talk, making sure that no one will disturb you and that you feel calm. Remember to show concern and compassion. Avoid judging the situation or the patients themselves. Do not make

accusations ("it's your fault, why did you lose weight, you could stop if you wanted to, it's just a matter of will," etc.). Do not stress your anger or irritation. Act as an educating, mature model. If you act with composure and respect, it is likely that the patient will do the same.

3. Use the rules of negotiating a contract for treatment, proper diet, and so forth. Try to negotiate daily portions of food to be eaten. Remember that, often overloaded with duties and perfectionist, the patient will strive to fully control the situation and meet all expectations, which can deepen the mental mechanisms of eating disorders.

4. In an ongoing dialog, make the patient start treatment as soon as possible. Disturbed eating behaviors become more difficult to treat with time. It is important that the person is examined by a doctor as soon as possible to assess whether he needs to be hospitalized or whether outpatient treatment will be sufficient. In some situations (e.g., when the BMI indicates malnutrition, when the patient displays very highly obsessive behaviors and thoughts about eating or losing weight or is unable to break the resulting vicious circle of destructive behaviors), the hospital brings relief and respite. Eating disorders can be fatal, and most patients are unable to properly assess their health and circumstances. Their fate often lies in the hands of their relatives and whether they recognize the signs and symptoms of eating disorders (e.g., hidden weight loss, artificial weight gain through lying, drinking large amounts of water, weighing down the body with heavy objects before weighing on a scale, etc.).

5. Make sure that the treatment is comprehensive from the very beginning, as it significantly increases its effectiveness. In addition to medical treatment (control of the somatic state), consider suggesting individual and/or family therapy, marriage counseling, or dietitian counseling.

6. If the patients are undergoing treatment, do not disturb them, do not be overprotective, and do not focus only on eating (do not watch over the patient's eating and do not talk about eating only), but start encouraging them to take responsibility for their actions (e.g., let them clean up after provoked vomiting, participate in replenishing food in the house after a binging episode). Do not try to overcontrol eating if body weight and other parameters related to the current physical condition are checked during treatment already. Any risks and threats will be communicated to you and will not be kept secret. One of the primary tasks of treatment is for the patients to learn how to control their own behavior, so let them keep trying and making mistakes until they learn it.

7. In everyday conversations, do not highlight topics related to appearance and body weight. Bringing attention to excessive thinness can be taken

as a compliment and will motivate further weight loss by acting as a reward.

8. Make the patients feel that their personality and psyche, not only the sphere of food and eating, matter for you as a parent. Respect their privacy as much as possible, especially with adolescent patients (e.g., do not check their personal correspondence, do not read their diaries, do not search their belongings, etc.). If you do, you risk losing the basis for trust between you. Without it, building the authority of an adult figure influencing the adolescent's identity is impossible.

9. As a parent, do not be obliged to feel sorry for the child – he may perceive it as pity, which will negatively affect his self-esteem. Feedback is needed which supports independence and autonomy. Avoid suggestions and so-called "common sense" advice (it immediately breeds opposition).

10. It might seem that your child/partner is being asked difficult personal questions in treatment. It is important that you remain in the role of the parent (partner) who supports these efforts (because they serve the same common goal of recovery). Do not worry that something is happening in treatment without your knowledge or that you are being criticized or blamed for the eating disorder. Therapy is about helping the whole family and supporting the parent's role in the adolescent's further development rather than about finding fault in the family and the therapist's authoritative role. Therapy serves the family, builds new possibilities, and corrects what is disturbed without destroying the bond between the parents and their children.

11. Try to remember that family life does not focus entirely on the person with an eating disorder and that they do not consciously take advantage of the so-called secondary benefits of the disorder (attention, forgiveness, less duties and responsibilities, etc.). The person with an eating disorder should be treated fairly as an equal.

Taking together the above psychological characteristics and the specificity of relationships in families of patients with eating disorders, it is worth pointing out that they may be important for planning the diagnosis and psychological therapy of patients with eating disorders experiencing body image distortions. During psychological therapy, it is important to support the family members in finding the so-called personal strengths (in emotions and behavior), so that they do not focus on guilt and helplessness, but rather support the development and healing of the person they love. There is no doubt that they want to do everything they can, and many actions they undertake are provoked by fear. The family creates a basic support system (especially when living with a person with an eating disorder). Therefore, it is important to strengthen new, healthy behaviors that the family will be able to model for the patient. It is also important for family members to learn about constructive coping strategies during this difficult situation.

Psychological and sociocultural profiles of body image in young women and men

The diagnosis and characterization of psychological profiles describing the specificity of sociocultural indicators of body image in young women and men are an important element in the psychological diagnosis of risk factors of body image distortions. These distortions may facilitate "anorexic readiness" or bigorexia. The results of many studies confirm the phenomenon of objectification (sexualization) of the body in women, and increasingly often in men, in western cultures (Fredrickson & Roberts, 1997; Izydorczyk et al., 2020; Manago et al., 2014; Rollero, 2012; Zurbriggen et al., 2011). Recent studies also emphasize the role of social media in shaping both women's (Monks et al., 2021) and men's (Gültzow et al., 2020) body image. The current cultural trends strengthen objectification of the body for both sexes, which is visible in the excessive pursuit of the sociocultural standards of attractiveness. At the same time, this pursuit contributes to negative overall self-esteem (Rollero, 2012; Zurbriggen et al., 2011). The increasing frequency of promoting the current body image standards in the media leads to perceived pressure and internalization of excessive striving for thinness and muscle tone (Fredrickson & Roberts, 1997; Izydorczyk et al., 2020; Rollero, 2012; Tiggemann et al., 2007; Zurbriggen et al., 2011). The significance of western sociocultural predictors of the female and male body image is explained by Thompson's multi-factor body image model (Thompson et al., 1999; Thornborrow et al., 2020; Tylka, 2011) and by Fredrickson and Roberts' (1997) sociocultural theory of body objectification.

In order to examine body image in healthy Polish women and men, and thus to indicate its specific psychological and sociocultural features, Izydorczyk et al. examined a population of 422 women and 776 men between 2017 and 2020. Body image was defined as a psychological structure comprised of the assessment of own appearance and attractiveness, satisfaction with own appearance overall, as well as with individual body parts, care for own appearance, assessment of own physical fitness, care for physical fitness, preoccupation with and anxiety related to obesity, frequency of monitoring own body weight, adherence to various diets, assessment of body weight, sense of health and care for health, and sensitivity to disease symptoms (Cash, 2004). Sociocultural standards of body image in the media were assumed to have a four-factor structure. The first factor was the level of internalization of sociocultural standards of body image and appearance promoted in the media. When internalized, they determine the attitude toward body image. The second factor was the level of pressure experienced due to the various body image-related information in the media. The third factor was the internalization of sociocultural standards of an athletic body shape (body musculature) promoted in the media. The fourth factor was the tendency to search for information about body image and appearance in the media (Izydorczyk & Lizińczyk, 2020).

The main inclusion criteria in the study were: informed consent and early adulthood (18–35 years). The exclusion criterion was the presence of mental and somatic disorders related to the body as well as currently undergoing various forms of treatment (psychotherapy). Data analysis was carried out by members of the research team (including graduate students) between 2017 and 2020 in several Polish cities, both online and face-to-face. The research project was approved by the Research Ethics Committee of the Institute of Applied Psychology, Faculty of Management and Social Communication, Jagiellonian University, Kraków. The *Multidimensional Body-Self Relations Questionnaire* (MBSRQ) by Thomas F. Cash (2004; Cash & Grasso, 2005) was used to measure the participants' body image. The questionnaire consists of 69 items assessing the emotional and cognitive aspects of body image. It includes nine scales: *self-classified weight* (SCW), *appearance orientation* (AO), *appearance evaluation* (AE), *body areas satisfaction scale* (BAS), *overweight preoccupation* (OP), *fitness orientation* (FO), *fitness evaluation* (FE), *heath evaluation* (HE), *health orientation* (HO), and *illness orientation* (IO). Answers are given on a five-point Likert scale. Mean scores were calculated for each scale. The higher the score, the greater the satisfaction with the body and its areas and functions. An exploratory factor analysis on a Polish sample of 341 women aged 18–35 years revealed a factor structure similar to the polish version of the MBSRQ (Brytek-Matera & Rogoza, 2015). Its internal consistency was assessed using the McDonald's omega coefficient and it ranged from 0.66 to 0.91.

The *Sociocultural Attitudes Towards Appearance Questionnaire* (SATAQ 3) by Thompson and Gray (1995), in the Polish adaptation by Izydorczyk and Lizińczyk (2020) was also used. Answers to the SATAQ 3 are given on a five-point Likert scale. Cronbach's α coefficients for the individual scales were as follows: *internalization–general* = 0.93, (Polish version = 0.91), *internalization–athlete* = 0.80 (Polish version = 0.96), *pressures* = 0.92 (Polish version = 0.78), and *information* = 0.96 (Polish version = 0.89).

In order to conduct a psychometric and clinical analysis of the results and to diagnose the inter- and intragroup differences in healthy Polish women and men, *k*-means cluster analysis was used. The distribution of selected clusters (sociocultural and psychological profiles) describing the participants' body image was analyzed. Cluster analysis groups the verified elements into relatively homogeneous groups (clusters) based on the similarity between the results on the independent variable, expressed by the similarity function (Hartigan & Wong, 1979). The analysis distinguished three clusters in the female sample and three clusters in the male sample. To carry out the cluster analysis, the variables were standardized. As a result, the scales of the questionnaires used in the study were unified. Scale values below 0 indicated lowered and low scores, while values above 0 indicated elevated and high scores. Significant differences between the three female and male clusters in terms of the indicated psychological and sociocultural profiles of body image were revealed (Figs. 2.1, 2.2.). The psychometric characteristics of these differences are presented in Table 2.1. Women (mean age = 23.18, BMI = 22.52) and men (mean age = 22.32, BMI = 23.70) were similar in terms of age and BMI. These variables allowed to define both groups as young, healthy (in terms of body weight) adults subject to the process of cultural westernization.

The statistical analysis (see Table 2.1) indicated differences on all variables (apart from sociocultural variables of internalization of sociocultural norms of body image, that is, internalization–general, information, as well as HO, that is, the commitment to a healthy lifestyle). Young women scored significantly higher than men on the following variables:

- appearance orientation (men reported significantly higher general satisfaction with the appearance of their body and its individual parts);
- overweight preoccupation, that is, fear of obesity, frequency of monitoring one's own body weight, and following diets;
- pressures: the perceived sociocultural and media pressure on body image standards.

On the other hand, men showed significantly higher FO, HO, and IO than women. Men also showed significantly higher internalization of sociocultural and media standards regarding the promotion of an athletic body shape (Internalization–athlete, see Table 2.1). The following section presents a psychological diagnosis of body image indices obtained via the cluster analysis.

Psychological and sociocultural characteristics of body image profiles in young women

The cluster analysis identified three clusters in the sample of 422 healthy young women. The clusters showed significant differences between on all psychological and sociocultural body image variables included in the study (see Table 2.2; Fig. 2.1). Cluster 1 comprised 102 women with BMI within the normal range, similar to women in the other two clusters. Cluster 1 was characterized by the highest and evenly distributed scores on the measured body image variables. The only below-average value in Cluster 1 was SCW.

Regarding OP, women in Cluster 1 scored significantly higher than women in Cluster 2, and significantly lower than women in Cluster 3. As for pressures and internalization, Cluster 1 included women with high scores on all related variables. They exhibited the highest (above the total sample mean) internalization–athlete scores. Accordingly, Cluster 1 was called the "athletic body image" profile. Cluster 2 comprised 148 women who exhibited the lowest (below the total sample mean) scores on all body image variables (except for SCW, similar to Cluster 1). At the same time, women in Cluster 2 exhibited the lowest scores on information,

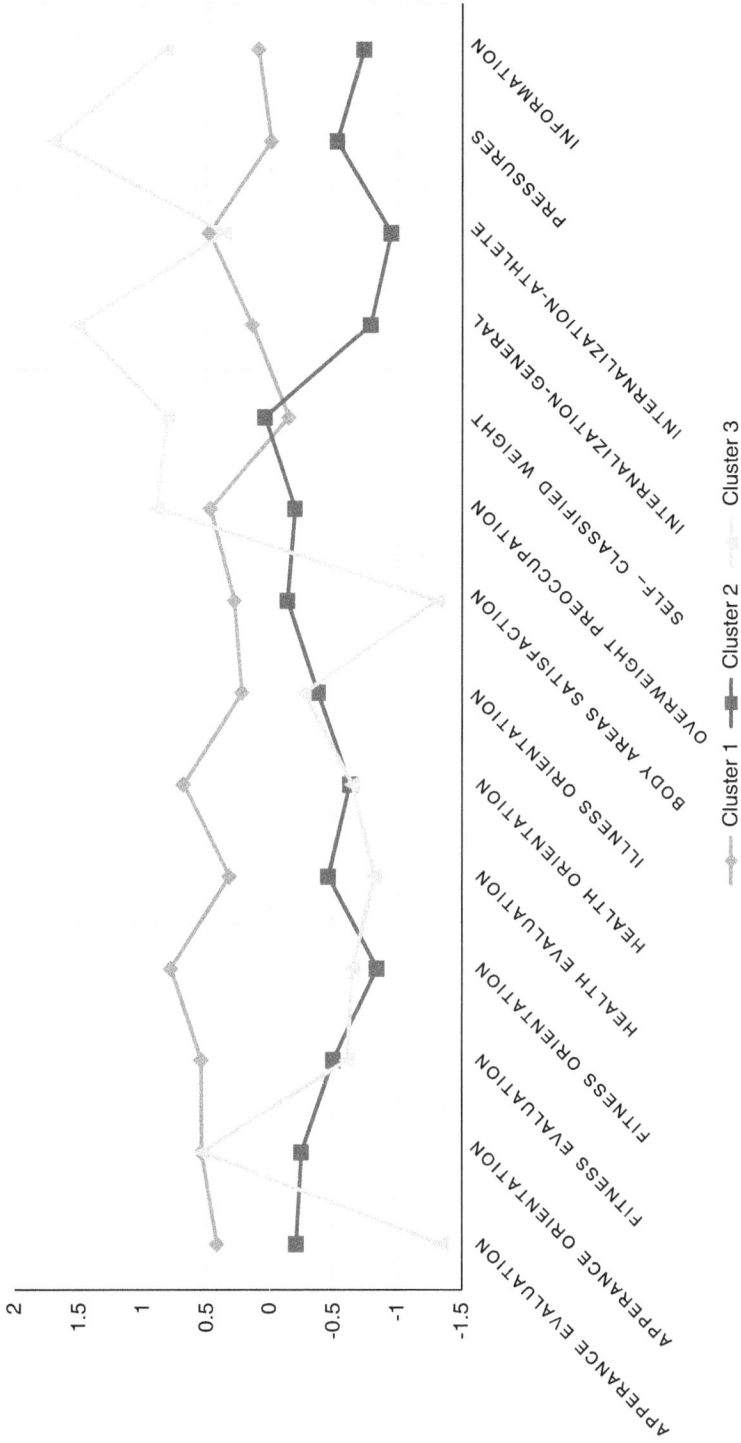

Figure 2.1 Scores on the individual body image variables in each of the clusters in the female sample (N = 422).

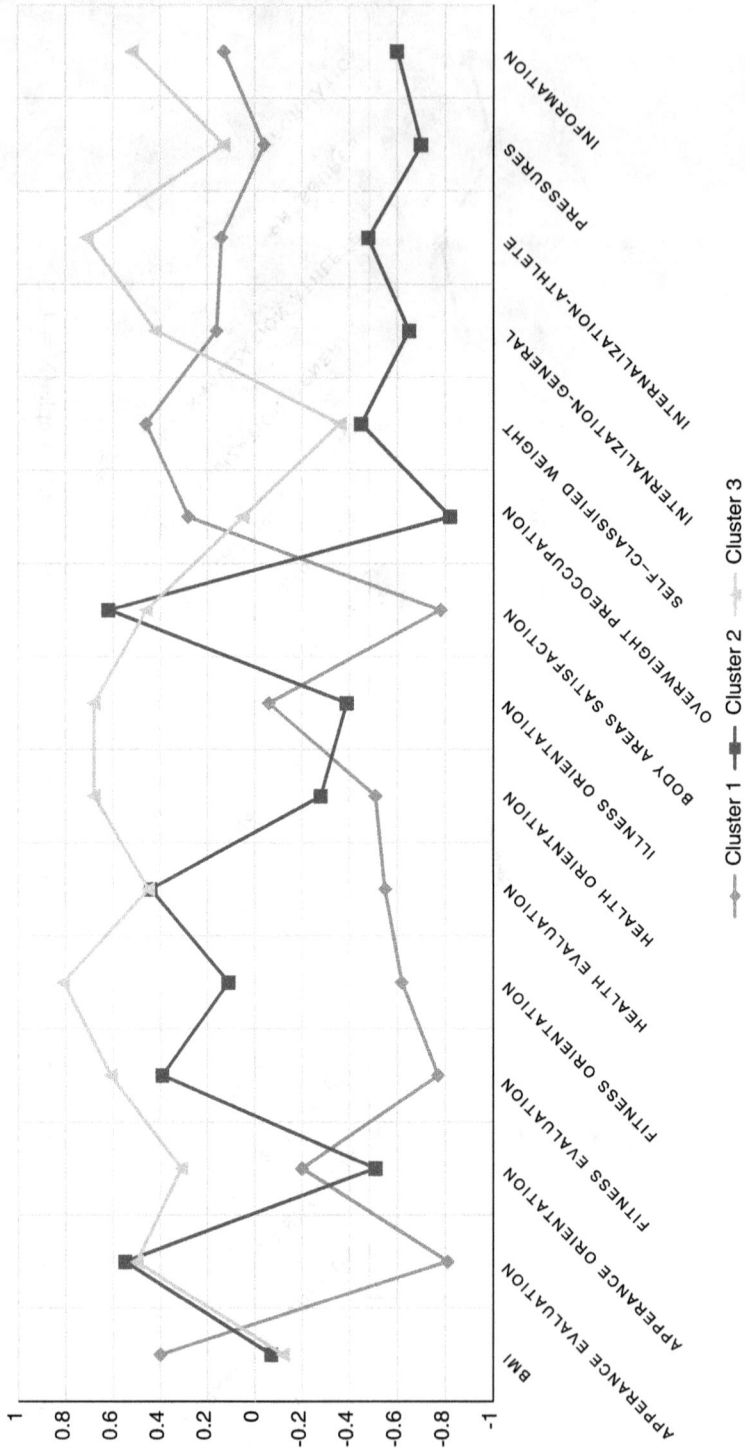

Figure 2.2 Scores on the individual body image variables in each of the clusters in the male sample (N = 766).

Table 2.1 Intergroup differences in psychological and sociocultural factors and body dissatisfaction (Mann–Whitney's *U* test for independent samples)

Variables	Women (N = 422)		Men (N = 776)		U	Z	p
	M	SD	M	SD			
AE	2.92	1.07	3.31	0.91	128,536	−6.15	.001
AO	3.45	0.74	3.21	0.71	133,368	5.31	.001
FE	3.02	1.06	3.34	1.03	136,060	−4.84	.001
FO	2.82	0.91	3.17	0.94	129,051	−6.06	.001
HE	3.21	0.85	3.58	0.82	122,521	−7.21	.001
HO	2.84	0.70	2.91	0.63	156,261	−1.31	.191
IO	2.78	0.62	2.96	0.77	103,146	−3.70	.001
BAS	3.06	0.78	3.39	0.73	123,878	−6.97	.001
OP	2.60	0.92	2.18	0.90	119,141	7.80	.001
SCW	3.20	0.73	2.96	0.77	132,867	5.40	.001
Internalization–general	22.80	9.89	21.78	7.52	159,104	0.81	.418
Internalization–athlete	12.54	4.93	13.85	4.54	137,018	−4.67	.001
Pressures	16.56	8.72	13.43	6.24	134,843	5.05	.001
Information	18.62	7.30	18.86	6.19	154,801	−1.56	.118

Note. MBSRQ subscales: AE = appearance evaluation; AO = appearance orientation; BAS = body areas satisfaction scale; FE = fitness evaluation; FO = fitness orientation; OP = overweight preoccupation; SCW = self-classified weight; HE = health evaluation; HO = health orientation; IO = illness orientation.

Table 2.2 Standardized mean values for the individual cluster scores on psychological and sociocultural variables and body dissatisfaction in women (N = 422)

Body image variables	Cluster 1 N = 102	Cluster 2 N = 148	Cluster 3 N = 92	df	F	p
BMI	−0.14	−0.29	−0.29	339	1.65	.194
AE	0.42	-0.21	−1.34	339	98.95	.001
AO	0.54	−0.25	0.54	339	27.10	.001
FE	0.54	−0.50	−0.61	339	50.92	.001
FO	0.78	−0.84	−0.65	339	170.54	.001
HE	0.32	−0.46	−0.82	339	41.52	.001
HO	0.68	−0.63	−0.65	339	80.56	.001
IO	0.22	−0.38	−0.27	339	17.53	.001
BAS	0.28	−0.14	−1.31	339	95.54	.001
OP	0.47	−0.20	0.89	339	42.10	.001
SCW	−0.15	0.04	0.81	339	31.26	.001
Internalization–general	0.14	−0.79	1.51	339	268.09	.001
Internalization–athlete	0.48	−0.95	0.36	339	119.00	.001
Pressures	−0.01	−0.53	1.69	339	225.69	.001
Information	0.09	−0.74	0.82	339	81.02	.001

Note. MBSRQ subscales: AE = appearance evaluation; AO = appearance orientation; BAS = body areas satisfaction scale; FE = fitness evaluation; FO = fitness orientation; OP = overweight preoccupation; SCW = self-classified weight; HE = health evaluation; HO = health orientation; IO = illness orientation.

pressures, and internalization–general (see Table 2.2; Fig. 2.1). Due to the highest OP scores, Cluster 2 was called the "body weight preoccupation" profile. Cluster 3 comprised 92 women who differed the most from the other women on all body image variables related to the sociocultural influence, especially pressures and internalization–general, as well as information. Only internalization–athlete scores were similar in strength to Cluster 1. Thus, Cluster 3 was called the "sociocultural" profile.

Psychological and sociocultural characteristics of body image profiles in young men

The cluster analysis also indicated three clusters in the sample of 776 healthy, young men. Significant differences between the clusters were confirmed in terms of all psychological and sociocultural variables included in the study (see Table 2.3; Fig. 2.2).

In the male sample, the cluster analysis identified three clusters which were much more differentiated than the female clusters. Cluster 1 included 205 men with the highest BMI value in the sample, low (significantly below the sample mean) AE and BAS, low FE, low FO, and low HO as well as high OF. Among the sociocultural variables, both internalization–general, internalization–athlete, and information were at a similar (above average) level. On the other hand, pressures scores were below the total sample mean. Thus, Cluster 1 was called the "low body self-esteem and high overweight fear" profile.

Table 2.3 Standardized mean values for the individual cluster scores on psychological and sociocultural variables and body dissatisfaction in men (N = 776)

Body image diagnostic indicators	Cluster 1 N = 205	Cluster 2 N = 148	Cluster 3 N = 28	d	F	p
BMI	0.40	−0.07	−0.12	698	15.67	.001
AE	−0.81	0.55	0.50	698	260.83	.001
AO	−0.20	−0.51	0.31	698	50.98	.001
FE	−0.77	0.39	0.61	698	188.29	.001
FO	−0.62	0.11	0.81	698	160.00	.001
HE	−0.55	0.44	0.45	698	95.00	.001
HO	−0.51	−0.28	0.68	698	139.40	.001
IO	−0.06	−0.39	0.68	698	80.74	.001
BAS	−0.78	0.62	0.46	698	222.23	.001
OP	0.28	−0.82	0.05	698	108.06	.001
SCW	0.46	−0.45	−0.36	698	63.28	.001
Internalization–general	0.16	−0.65	0.42	698	144.66	.001
Internalization–athlete	0.14	−0.48	0.71	698	129.44	.001
Pressures	−0.04	−0.70	0.13	698	97.11	.001
Information	0.13	−0.60	0.52	698	125.18	.001

Note. MBSRQ subscales: AE = appearance evaluation; AO = appearance orientation; BAS = body areas satisfaction scale; FE = fitness evaluation; FO = fitness orientation; OP = overweight preoccupation; SCW = self-classified weight; HE = health evaluation; HO = health orientation; IO = illness orientation.

Cluster 2 was made up of 248 men with the lowest BMI in the male sample, simultaneously showing high (significantly above the total sample mean) AE and BAS, as well as high HE, FE, and FO, with lower HO and IO. Men in Cluster 2 also showed low (significantly below the total sample mean) OP and SAW. All the sociocultural variables included in the study were the lowest in the total sample, which would suggest the lowest level of internalization and pressures regarding body image standards. Thus, Cluster 2 was named the "high body satisfaction, physical fitness, and health with low overweight fear" profile.

Cluster 3 comprised 248 men with BMIs similar to men from Cluster 2 (lower than Cluster 1). These men reported the highest scores on body image variables in the entire male sample, showing a high level of AE and BAS, AO, FE, and FO. At the same time, men in this cluster showed below-average OP. Compared with the total male sample, men in Cluster 3 also achieved the highest scores on the sociocultural variables, including internalization–athlete. Thus, Cluster 3 was titled the "strong internalization of sociocultural standards, very high body, physical fitness, and health satisfaction, and low overweight" profile.

References

Arroyo A., & Segrin, C. (2013). Family interactions and disordered eating attitudes: The mediating roles of social competence and psychological distress. *Communication Monographs*, *80*(4), 399–424. 10.1080/03637751.2013.828158

Balottin, L., Mannarini, S., Rossi, M., Rossi, G., & Balottin, U. (2017). The parental bonding in families of adolescents with anorexia: Attachment representations between parents and offspring. *Neuropsychiatric Disease and Treatment*, *13*, 319–327. 10.2147/NDT.S128418

Bowlby, J. (1988). *Secure base. Clinical applications of attachment theory*. Routledge.

Bowlby, J. (2021). *Przywiązanie [Attachment]*. Wydawnictwo Naukowe PWN.

Bowlby, J., & Ainsworth, M. D. S. (1965). *Child care and the growth of love* (2nd ed.). Penguin Books.

Brytek-Matera, A. (2008). *Obraz ciała-obraz siebie. Wizerunek własnego ciała w ujęciu psychospołecznym* [Body image and self image. Body image in the psycho-social approach]. Difin.

Brytek-Matera, A., & Rogoza, R. (2015). Validation of the Polish version of the Multidimensional Body-Self Relations Questionnaire among women. *Eating and Weight Disorders*, *20*(1), 109–117. 10.1007/s40519-014-0156-x

Cash, T. F. (2004). Body image: Past, present, and future. *Body Image*, *1*(1), 1–5. 10.1016/S1740-1445(03)00011-1

Cash, T. F. (2012). Cognitive-behavioral perspectives on body image. In T. F. Cash (Ed.), *Encyclopedia of body image and human appearance* (pp. 334–342). Academic Press.

Cash, T. F., & Grasso, K. (2005). The norms and stability of new measures of the multidimensional body image construct. *Body Image*, *2*(2), 199–203. 10.1016/j.bodyim.2005.03.007

Cash, T. F., & Pruzinsky T. (Eds.). (2004). *Body image. A handbook of theory, research, and clinical practice* (pp. 235–242). The Guilford Press.

Cerniglia, L., Cimino, S., & Tafà, M. E. M. P. (2017). Family profiles in eating disorders: Family functioning and psychopathology. *Psychology Research and Behavior Management*, *10*, 305–312. 10.2147/PRBM.S145463

Domene, J. & Socholotiuk, K. D., & Young, R. A. (2011). The early stages of the transition to adulthood: Similarities and differences between mother-daughter and mother-son dyads. *Journal of Qualitative Research in Psychology*, *8*(3), 273–291. 10.1080/14780880903568022

Enten, R. S., & Golan, M. (2009). Parenting styles and eating disorder pathology. *Appetite*, *52*(3), 784–787. 10.1016/j.appet.2009.02.013

Fonagy, P., Gergely, G., & Target, M. (2007). The parent-infant dyad and the construction of the subjective self. *Journal of Child Psychology and Psychiatry and Allied Disciplines*, *48*(3–4), 288–328.

Fonagy, P., Luyten, P., & Bateman, A. (2015). Translation: Mentalizing as treatment target in borderline personality disorder. *Personality Disorders: Theory, Research, and Treatment*, *6*(4), 380–392. 10.1037/per0000113

Fonagy, P., Luyten, P., Bateman, A., Gergely, G., Strathearn, L., Target, M., & Allison, E. (2013). Przywiązanie a patologia osobowości [Attachment and personality pathology]. In J. F. Clarkin, P. Fonagy, & G.O. Gabbard (Eds.), *Psychoterapia psychodynamiczna zaburzeń osobowości* [Psychodynamic psychotherapy of personality disorders] (pp. 61–119). Wydawnictwo Uniwersystetu Jagiellońskiego.

Franzoni, S. K., & Shields, S. A. (1984). The Body Esteem Scale: Multidimensional structure and sex differences in a college population. *Journal of Personality Assessment*, *48*(2), 173–178. 10.1207/s15327752jpa4802_12

Fredrickson, B. L., & Roberts T. A. (1997). Objectification theory. Toward understanding women's lived experiences and mental health risks. *Psychology of Women Quarterly*, 21(2), 173–206. 10.1111/j.1471-6402.1997.tb00108.x

Gander, M., Sevecke, K., & Buchheim, A. (2015). Eating disorders in adolescence: Attachment issues from a developmental perspective. *Frontiers in Psychology*, *6*, 11366. 10.3389/fpsyg.2015.01136

Garner, D. M. (2004). *EDI-3. Eating Disorders Inventory. Professional Manual.* Psychological Assessment Resources, Inc.

Glickauf-Hughes Ch., & Wells M. (1997). *Object relations psychotherapy. An individual and integreative approach to diagnosis and treatment.* Jason Aronson, Inc.

Głowacka, N. (2020). Nauczyliśmy się tego od rąk, które nas kiedyś otaczały: - związek dotyku i relacji z rodzicami i obrazem ciała. In K. Schier (Ed.), *Samotne ciało* [The lonely body] (pp. 17–39). Wydawnictwo Scholar.

Gültzow, T., Guidry, J. P. D., Schneider, F., & Hoving, C. (2020). Male body image portrayals on Instagram. *Cyberpsychology, Behavior, and Social Networking*, *23*, 281–289. 10.1089/cyber.2019.0368.

Hartigan J. A., & Wong M. A. (1979). A k-means clustering algorithm. *Journal of the Royal Statistical Society: Series C (Applied Statistics)*, *28*(1), 100–108. 10.2307/2346830

Iniewicz, G., Józefik, B., Namysłowska, I., & Ulasińska, R. (2002). Obraz relacji rodzinnych w oczach pacjentek chorujących na anoreksję psychiczną - częśc II

[The subjective picture of family relations in female anorexia patients – Part II].
Psychiatria Polska, *1*, 65–81.

Izydorczyk, B. (2010). Psychoterapia oparta na teorii relacji z obiektem i psychodramie: integracyjne podejście w leczeniu zaburzeń odżywiania. [Object relations- and psychodrama-based psychotherapy: An integrative approach to the treatment of eating disorders]. *Psychiatria Polska*, *44*(5), 677–691.

Izydorczyk, B., & Lizińczyk, S. (2020). The Polish adaptation of the sociocultural attitudes towards appearance SATAQ 3 questionnaire. *Health Psychology Report*, *8*(1), 68–82. 10.5114/hpr.2020.91443

Izydorczyk, B., & Sitnik-Warchulska, K. (2018). Sociocultural appearance standards and risk factors for eating disorders in adolescents and women of various ages. *Frontiers in Psychology*, *9*(429), 1–21. 10.3389/fpsyg.2018.00429

Izydorczyk, B., Sitnik-Warchulska, K., Lizińczyk, S., & Lipowska, M. (2020). Socio-cultural standards promoted by the mass media as predictors of restrictive and bulimic behavior. *Frontiers in Psychiatry*, *11*(506), 1–14. 10.3389/fpsyt.2020.00506

Johns, A., & Peters, L. (2012). Self-discrepancies and the situational domains of social phobia. *Behaviour Change*, *29*(2), 109–125. 10.1017/bec.2012.1

Józefik, B. (Ed.) (1999). *Anoreksja i bulimia psychiczna. Rozumienie i leczenie zaburzeń odżywiania się* [Anorexia and bulimia. Understanding and treatment of eating disorders]. Wydawnictwo Uniwersytetu Jagiellońskiego.

Józefik, B. (2014). *Kultura, ciało, (nie)jedzenie* [Culture, body, (not)eating]. Wydawnictwo Uniwersytetu Jagiellońskiego.

Józefik, B., Iniewicz, G., Namysłowska, I., & Ulasińska, R. (2002). Obraz relacji rodzinnych w oczach pacjentek chorujących na anoreksję psychiczną – część I [The subjective picture of family relations in female anorexia patients – Part I]. *Psychiatria Polska*, *1*, 51–64.

Józefik, B., Iniewicz, G., & Ulasińska, R. (2010). Wzory przywiązania, samoocena i płeć psychologiczna w anoreksji i bulimii psychicznej [Attachment patterns, self-esteem, and psychological gender in anorexia and bulimia]. *Psychiatria Polska*, *44*(5), 665–676.

Kearney-Cooke A. (2002). Familial influences on body image development. In T. F. Cash, & T. Pruzinsky (Eds.), *Body image: A handbook of theory, research, and clinical practice* (pp. 99–107). Guilford Press.

Krueger, D. W. (2002a). Psychodynamic perspective on body image. In T. F. Cash, & T. Pruzinsky (Eds.), *Body image. A handbook of theory, research, and clinical practice* (pp. 30–37). The Guilford Press.

Krueger, D. W. (2002b). *Integrating body self and psychological self. Creating a new story in psychoanalysis and psychotherapy*. Bruner-Routledge.

Lipowska, M, & Lipowski, M. (2013). Polish normalization of the Body Esteem Scale. *Health Psychology Report*, *1*, 72–81. 10.5114/hpr.2013.40471

Manago, A. M., Ward, L. M., Lemm, K. M., Reed, L., & Seabrook, R. (2014). Facebook involvement, objectified body consciousness, body shame, and sexual assertiveness in college women and men. *Sex Roles 72*(1-2), 1–14. 10.1007/s11199-014-0441-1

Matczak, A. (2007). KKS - Kwestionariusz Kompetencji Społecznych [KSS – Social Competences Questionnaire]. *Pracownia testów Psychologicznych Polskiego Towarzystwa Psychologicznego*. Warszawa Pracownia Testów Psychologicznych.

Monks, H., Costello, L., Dare, J., & Boyd, E.R. (2021). "We're continually comparing ourselves to something": Navigating body image, media, and social media ideals at the nexus of appearance, health, and wellness. *Sex Roles, 84*, 221–237. 10.1007/s11199-020-01162

Monteleone, A. M., Ruzzi, V., Patriciello, G., Pellegrino, F., Cascino, G., Castellini, G., Steardo, L., Monteleone, P., & Maj, M. (2019). Parental bonding, childhood maltreatment and eating disorder psychopathology: An investigation of their interactions. *Eating and Weight Disorders, 25*(3), 577–589. 10.1007/s40519-019-00649-0

Moretti, M. M., & Higgins, E. T. (1990). The development of self-system vulnerabilities: Social and cognitive factors in developmental psychopathology. In R. J. Sternberg, & J. Kolligian Jr. (Eds.). *Competence considered* (pp. 286–314). Yale University Press.

Moretti, M. M., & Higgins, E.T. (1999). Own versus other standpoints in self-regulation: Developmental antecedents and functional consequences. *Review of General Psychology, 3*(3),188–223. 10.1037/1089-2680.3.3.188

Niewiadomska, I., Kulik, A., & Hajduk, A. (2005). *Jedzenie. Uzależenienia: fakty i mity*. [Eating. Addictions: Facts and myths]. Wydawnictwo Gaudium

O'Connor, C. L. (2000). *Body image disturbance in relation to self-perceptions of physical attractiveness, social competence, and need for approval in college women* [Doctoral dissertation, University of Windsor]. Electronic Theses and Dissertations. http://scholar.uwindsor.ca/etd/1318

Ostoja-Zawadzka, K. (1999). Cykl życia rodziny [The family life cycle]. In B. de Barbaro (Ed.), *Wprowadzenie do systemowej terapii rodzin* [Introduction to family systems therapy] (pp.18–30). Wydawnictwo Uniwersytetu Jagiellońskiego.

Parker, G. (1998). *Parental Bonding Instrument. Annotated bibliography of PBI*. Black Dog Institute.

Parker, G., Tupling, H., & Brown, L. B. (1979). A parental bonding instrument. *British Journal of Medical Psychology, 52*(1), 1–10. 10.1111/j.2044-8341 .1979.tb02487

Patton, S. C., Beaujen, A. A., & Benedict, H. E. (2014). Parental bonds, attachment anxiety, media susceptibility, and body dissatisfaction: A mediation model. *Developmental Psychology, 50*(8), 2124–2133. 10.1037/a0037111

Popiel, A., & Praglowska, E. (2006). Terapia poznawczo- behawioralna schizofrenii. In J. Meder (Ed.), *Oddziaływania psychologiczne w schizofrenii* (s. 31–43). Warszawa: Biblioteka Psychiatrii Polskiej.

Rollero, Ch. (2012). Men and women facing objectification: The effects of media models on well-being, self-esteem and ambivalent sexism. *International Journal of Social Psychology, 28*(3), 373–382. 10.1174/021347413807719166

Sakson-Obada, O. (2009a). *Pamięć ciała. Ja cielesne w relacji przywiązania i w traumie* [The body's memory. The body Self in attachment relationships and trauma]. Wydawnictwo Difin.

Sakson-Obada, O. (2009b). Trauma jako czynnik ryzyka dla zaburzeń Ja cielesnego [trauma as a risk factor for the disorders of the bodily ego]. *Przegląd Psychologiczny, 52*(3), 309–326.

Salcuni, S., Parolin, L., & Colli, A. (2017). Attachment research and eating disorders: A measurement perspective-literature review. *Polskie Forum Psychologiczne, 22*(3), 478–504. 10.14656/PFP20170308

Schier, K. (2010). *Piękne brzydactwo. Psychologiczna problematyka obrazu ciała i jego zaburzeń* [Ugly beauty. The psychology of body image and its disorders]. Wydawnictwo Naukowe Scholar.

Schier, K. (2020). *Samotne ciało* [The lonely body]. Wydawnictwo Scholar.

Sepúlveda, A. R., Lacruz, T., Solano, S., Blanco, M., Moreno, A., Rojo, M., Beltrán, L. & Graell, M. (2020). Identifying loss of control eating within childhood obesity: The importance of family environment and child psychological distress. *Children, 7*(11), 225. 10.3390/children7110225

Strauman T. J., & Higgins E. T. (1988). Self-discrepancies as predictors of vulnerability to distinct syndromes of chronic emotional distress. *Journal of Personality, 56*(4), 685–707. 10.1111/j.1467-6494.1988.tb00472.x

Tantleff-Dunn S., & Gokee J. L. (2002). Interpersonal influences on body image development. In T. F. Cash, & T. Pruzinsky (Eds.), *Body image. A handbook of theory, research, and clinical practice* (pp. 108–117). The Guilford Press.

Tasca, G. A. (2019). Attachment and eating disorders: A research update. *Current Opinion in Psychology, 25*, 59–64. 10.1016/j.copsyc.2018.03.003

Tasca, G. A., & Balfour, L. (2014). Attachment and eating disorders: A review of current research. *International Journal of Eating Disorders, 47*(7), 710–717. 10.1002/eat.22302

Tasca, G. A., Szadkowski, L., Illing, V., Trinneer, A., Grenon, R., Demidenko, N., Krysanski, V., Balfour, L., & Bissada, H. (2009). Adult attachment, depression, and eating disorder symptoms: The mediating role of affect regulation strategies. *Personality and Individual Differences, 47*(6), 662–667. 10.1016/j.paid.2009.06.006

Tetley, A., Moghaddam, N. G., Dawson, D. L., & Rennoldson, M. (2014). Parental bonding and eating disorders: A systematic review. *Eating Behaviors, 15*(1), 49–59. 10.1016/j.eatbeh.2013.10.008

Thompson, J. K., Heinberg, L. J., Altabe, M., & Tantleff-Dunn, S. (1999). *Exacting beauty: Theory, assessment and treatment of body image disturbance.* American Psychological Association.

Thompson, M. A., & Gray, J. J. (1995). Development and validation of a new body-image assessment scale. *Journal of Personality Assessment, 64*(2), 258–269. 10.1207/s15327752jpa6402_6

Thornborrow, T., Onwuegbusi, T., Mohamed, S., Boothroyd, L. G., & Tovée, M. J. (2020). Muscles and the media: A natural experiment across cultures in men's body image. *Frontiers in Psychology, 11*, 495. 10.3389/fpsyg.2020.00495

Tiggemann, M., Martins, Y., & Kirkbride, A. (2007). Oh to be lean and muscular: Body image ideals in gay and heterosexual men. *Psychology of Men & Masculinity, 8*(1), 15–24. 10.1037/1524-9220.8.1.15

Treasure, J., Todd, G. (2016). Interpersonal maintaining factors in eating disorder: Skill sharing interventions for carers. In Y. Latzer, & D. Stein (Eds.), *Bio-psycho-social contributions to understanding eating disorders* (pp. 125–137). Springer International Publishing.

Tylka, T. L. (2011). Refinement of the tripartite influence model for men: Dual body image pathways to body change behaviors. *Body Image, 8*(3), 199–207. 10.1016/j.bodyim.2011.04.008

Uzunian, L. G., & de Souza Vitalle, M. S. (2015). Social skills: A factor of protection against eating disorders in adolescents. *Ciência & Saúde Coletiva, 20*(11), 3495–3508. 10.1590/1413-812320152011.18362014

Wertheim, E. H., Paxton, S. J., & Blaney, S. (2004). Risk factors for the development of body image disturbances. In J. K. Thompson (Ed.), *Handbook of eating disorders and obesity* (pp. 463–494). John Wiley & Sons.

Zurbriggen, E. L., Ramsey, L. R., & Jaworski, B. K. (2011). Self- and partner-objectification in romantic relationships: associations with media consumption and relationship satisfaction. *Sex Roles, 64*(7–8), 449–462. 10.1007/s11199-011-9933-4

3 Mental trauma and body image in eating disorders

The role of traumatic events, especially relational traumas, in eating disorders should be considered as an important point in the process of psychological diagnosis and psychotherapy of eating disorders. Documenting, based on the literature, the role of trauma in the development of body image disorders and anti-health eating behaviors, the author presents the results of their own research showing a relationship between the deficits in the secure attachment style (the presence of various situations of emotional deficits and emotional abandonment by caregivers in childhood) and the occurrence of restrictive eating behaviors in women with restrictive anorexia as well as the relationship between the experience of sexual and physical abuse and bulimic behaviors among women with bulimia and bulimic anorexia.

In order to conduct a psychological diagnosis of risk factors for the development of eating disorders in adults, the psychological measurement of the type and impact of experienced traumatic events must be taken into account both via the clinical interview as well as one or more diagnostic tools. Traumatic events include traffic accidents, natural and man-made disasters, psychological violence (including emotional deficits in the childhood bond), and physical and sexual violence. Searching for relationships between broadly understood mental trauma and body image distortions is very important for the process of diagnosis and treatment of eating disorders. Mental trauma is indicated in contemporary literature as an important factor influencing body image formation and experience (Izydorczyk, 2017b; Sakson-Obada, 2009a, 2009b; Skrzypska & Suchańska, 2011) as well as the development of eating disorder symptoms (Caslini et al., 2016; Collins et al., 2014; Franzoni et al., 2013; Hartt & Waller, 2002; Hewett, 2015; Kent & Waller, 2000; Kent et al., 1999; Madowitz et al., 2015; Moulton et al., 2015; McCormack et al., 2014; Racine & Wildes, 2015; Schier, 2020; Tahilani, 2015; Tasca et al., 2013).

According to Greenspan's (2000) theory of mind, the mind is formed in early childhood and is based on the quality of the relationship pattern with the primary caregiver. The developing mentalization of internal states (their expression through the mind) is influenced by emotional regulation and related bodily processes. Traumas "stored in the body" in patients with psychosomatic disorders (such as eating disorders) constitute a special type

DOI: 10.4324/9781003251088-3

of relationship between the body and the psyche (Schier, 2020). Among the specific types of psychological trauma related to the development of eating disorder symptoms are various childhood traumas experienced in relationships with other people, especially caregivers, significant others, and other adults. The traumas in question can be defined as the so-called relational traumas, associated with the experience of chronic emotional deficits, abandonment, and various forms of violence. In object relations theory, traumatic events, emotional deficits, and destructive object relationships, especially during childhood, are significant risk factors for eating disorders, as internalized, destructive patterns of relationships with a given object (guardian/parent) are reproduced in future relationships (Glickauf-Hughes & Wells, 1997). In light of attachment theory, emotional and cognitive patterns of functioning and relationships with others are based on early childhood relations with the primary caregiver (parent).

Shaped during socialization and upbringing, the insecure relationship pattern between the traumatized child and the primary caregiver maintains an anxious or anxious–avoidant attachment pattern later in life and leads to uncertainty in interpersonal relationships – common in patients with eating disorders (Izydorczyk, 2015a; Józefik, 2008; Józefik et al., 2010; Schier, 2020). The child and his body experiencing interpersonal trauma lack a soothing, internalized parental object on the body level and thus remain "alone" with his symptoms (Schier, 2020). Krystal (1977, 1979, 2000) distinguished two types of early childhood traumas: type I (one-time traumatic event, e.g., related to leaving the child unattended and endangering his life or health) and type II, that is, the cumulative impact of chronic traumatic events, for example, separation from the caregiver due to abandonment or hospitalization, lack of safety, neglect, physical violence, cold or emotionally unstable behaviors toward the child, excessive control and interference in his body through corporal punishment, or sexual abuse. Type II trauma is also termed relational or attachment trauma (Rzeszutek & Schier, 2008). Krystal's concept of trauma is related to Schur's theory of the development of psychosomatic disorders (Luban-Plozza et al., 1995; McDougall, 2014).

In addition to psychoanalytical theories explaining the development of psychosomatic disorders based on distortions of affective states due to attachment deficits, Fonagy's mentalization theory (Fonagy et al., 2007, 2013, 2015) offers a related account. According to Fonagy, distortions in the mentalization of one's own and others internal states may be the source of both personality disorders as well as eating disorders (Fonagy et al., 2007, 2013, 2015; Greenspan, 2000). Some Polish studies have indicated the impact of physical and sexual violence in shaping body experience. Chronic interpersonal trauma in early childhood is associated with disturbances in the body Self (Sakson-Obada, 2009a, 2009b). According to Krystal, this involves relational trauma, often centered around psychological, physical, or sexual violence. Relational trauma is based on disturbances in the early relationship with the caregiver and it inhibits establishing relationships with others later in life (Sakson-Obada, 2008, 2009a, 2009b). Victims of sexual trauma (especially from a significant other) often develop the so-called "traumatic bond with the aggressor," which is directly connected with disturbances in body experience (Skrzypska & Suchańska, 2011). Theoretical studies of interpersonal trauma (psychological, sexual and physical, and involving separation from the parents) indicate the traumatic bond as an important risk factor for self-harming behaviors (Kubiak & Sakson-Obada, 2016).

Regarding the importance of the emotional bond in the development of anorexia or psychological bulimia, it is also worth noting Krueger's (2002a, 2002b) theory of the development and pathology of the Self structure. This psychoanalytic theory also posits that patients with eating disorders have an inhibited sense of bodily boundaries related to emotional childhood experiences in the relationship with the primary caregiver (parent). Not having experienced, an emotional connection and an empathetic response to their childhood needs may cause difficulties in building appropriate psychological boundaries between one's own body and the outside world. According to Krueger (2002a, 2002b), the basic assumption about the role of the psychological bond in shaping the specificity of the body Self structure is consistent with the object relations approach to body image disorders. The specificity of the emotional connection forms the blueprint for the experiences of body image and physical experience. This is particularly important in the development of eating disorders, where the pattern of social relationships is impacted by difficulties in establishing an emotional bond, which may be rooted in prior relational trauma. The author's own research conducted in 2007–2012 (Izydorczyk, 2015b) on a population of 120 women with eating disorders receiving psychological therapy showed that they have experienced psychological trauma (Izydorczyk, 2017a). This may suggest a mutual relationship between psychological trauma and the development of symptoms of eating disorders. The research in question included women aged 20–26 years, suffering from anorexia (40%, BMI = 17.8), bulimia (30%, BMI = 20.63), and binge eating disorder (30%, BMI = 24.3). The research was conducted in centers for the treatment of anxiety disorders and eating disorders, where, during interviews and therapy sessions, the women indicated the presence of various traumatic events in their lives:

1. single recalled event from childhood and/or adolescence (accidents, catastrophes, difficult situations related to being left unattended, and risks to life or health);
2. single recalled event from adulthood (accidents, catastrophes, other various difficult situations with traumatic features);
3. various relational traumas during childhood and adolescence, that is, physical violence, sexual violence, separation from the caregiver, loss of a significant other, separation due to hospitalization, neglect,

emotionally cold or unstable behavior of the caregiver, abuse through corporal punishment, excessive control, and so forth.

4.   mental, physical, and/or sexual violence experienced in adulthood.

The sensitive data were obtained with the personal consent of each participant and covered by professional secrecy. The data were not included in the documentation accessible by other medical staff (except for the participants' physicians and psychotherapists). The frequency of the traumatic events was measured on a four-point scale. It was found that the self-reports of traumatic events and their duration (type of injury, duration, and repeatability) constitute sufficient data for empirical analysis. Selected categories of structured clinical interviews and data from the medical history of the surveyed women were also used to measure BMI, sociodemographic data (age, gender, place of residence, marital status), and the presence of the following medical diagnoses according to ICD-10 criteria: bulimia (F50.2), anorexia (F50.1), and overeating associated with other psychological disturbances (F50.4; F50.81 according to 2020 ICD-10 codes).

Garner's *Eating Disorder Inventory* (EDI; Polish adaptation: Żechowski, 2008; Garner, 2004; Izydorczyk, 2015a, 2015b) was used to measure psychological traits in the participants diagnosed with eating disorders. In this study, 120 women with eating disorders (clinical group) and 120 healthy women (without eating disorders and not receiving treatment for other mental disorders and diseases related to body image distortions; control group) were examined. The clinical group was further divided into two subgroups:

1.   women who experienced a single traumatic event in the past (including both accidents and catastrophes as well as instances of abandonment by caregivers, e.g., due to hospitalization).

2.   women who are currently suffering from long-term relational traumas which began both in childhood/adolescence or in adulthood.

The results (see Izydorczyk, 2017a) indicated that women with eating disorders who experienced single episode of traumatic events presented higher perfectionism and body dissatisfaction than women who experienced/were experiencing sexual and physical violence. The levels of distrust and uncertainty in building bonds and relationships with others was similar in both subgroups. Therefore, analyzing the differences in perfectionism between the participants, one may wonder whether its levels in the subgroups of women who experienced traumatic events is associated with restrictive patterns of behavior in relationships. The usually strong and excessive self-control that manifests itself through perfectionism may be a way of coping with the experienced deprivation of the sense of security and emotional closeness by a patient with an eating disorder (especially anorexia). In turn, this deprivation always results from traumatic events involving premature separation from the primary caregiver.

Women who experienced single traumatic event involving emotional abandonment by caregivers during childhood also showed increased perfectionism, which may correlate with increased restrictiveness characteristic of anorexic symptoms and constitute an unconscious response to the perceived emotional deprivation in early childhood (Izydorczyk, 2017a). The increased need for perfectionism in eating disorders can foster a sense of omnipotence and denial of the need for closeness. The subgroup of women who reported premature separation and emotional abandonment by one of the parents comprised no women who experienced traumatic events consisting of a direct attack on the body by another person (physical or sexual violence). Relational trauma involving physical and sexual violence was significant in the second subgroup of women, who mainly manifested symptoms of bulimia and binge eating disorder (Izydorczyk, 2017a). Women with eating disorders who experienced emotional abandonment in their childhood experienced the object/caregiver's "disappearance" rather than a direct assault on the body, as is often in the case with physical or sexual violence. Women with eating disorders who experienced relational trauma (mental, physical, or sexual violence) also had a greater intensity of bulimic (impulsive) tendencies than women with eating disorders who declared the presence of traumatic events in their lives consisting mainly of emotional abandonment (i.e., the first subgroup, see Table 3.1).

A Mann-Whitney's *U* comparison between the studied variables showed significant differences between women with eating disorders who experienced relational trauma in their lives (especially in childhood and adolescence) and those who did not. The former group exhibited significantly higher bulimic thinking and a tendency toward excessive, uncontrolled,

Table 3.1 Means of selected psychological traits in women with eating disorders, taking into account relational trauma (N = 120)

Psychological features	Women who have experienced a single traumatic event	Women who have experienced relational trauma	U	Z	p
Body dissatisfaction	13.92	16.26	1041.0	−1.345	.179
Interoceptive awareness	10.95	11.67	1138.0	−0.735	.462
Maturity fears	14.90	17.22	1036.0	−1.376	.169
Bulimia	16.16	17.48	850.0	−2.545	.011
Ineffectiveness	15.03	15.37	1218.0	−0.233	.816
Perfectionism	17.33	17.74	1075.5	−1.128	.259
Interpersonal distrust	10.44	9.87	1254.5	0.003	.997
Drive for thinness	17.33	17.70	1080.0	−1.126	.256

Source: Table reprinted from Izydorczyk, B. (2017a). Trauma in relation to psychological characteristics in women with eating disorders. Current Issues in Personality Psychology, 5(4), 244–259. https://doi.org/10.5114/cipp.2017.67047

and impulsive behavior toward food and eating (induced vomiting and other forms of purging).

The remaining psychological features remained at a similar and not statistically significant level between the two subgroups. Thus, tendencies toward bulimic and impulsive patterns of thinking, experiencing, and reacting may be greater in patients with eating disorders who have experienced psychological, sexual, and/or physical abuse. It can be hypothesized that bulimic tendencies and impulsivity in women with eating disorders may be an emotional response to the violation of bodily boundaries that takes place during relational trauma (physical or sexual violence). Impulsive bulimic symptoms are self-harming behaviors toward the body. It should be considered whether the bulimic symptom (provoked vomiting, other forms of purging, compulsive overeating) represents a specific, unconscious pattern of identification with the role of the aggressor. Women with bulimic and impulsive tendencies unconsciously violate the boundaries of their own body, as did the perpetrator of the relational trauma toward them.

The results of Izydorczyk (2015a, 2015b) also indicated that women diagnosed with bulimia and bulimic anorexia reported experiencing relational trauma (psychological, physical, and/or sexual violence) during childhood and adolescence significantly more often than women with restrictive anorexia. Only 7.4% of the women from the latter group reported experiencing relational trauma. Similarly, women with bulimia and binge eating disorder reported having experienced relational trauma.

Summarizing the above results, it can be said that women with bulimia and binge eating and purging anorexia reported experiencing relational trauma significantly more often. Women with restrictive anorexia did not report relational trauma, but they more often indicated the presence of emotional deficits, insecurity, emotional situations, and real abandonment in childhood and/or adolescence. How to understand this phenomenon? First, it may result from the limitations of the study itself and the sample (it may not have included participants diagnosed with restrictive anorexia who also experienced trauma during the preverbal period; Izydorczyk, 2017a; Sakson-Obada, 2009a, 2009b). According to psychoanalytic theories, the development of psychological anorexia often involves the experience of early childhood (preverbal period) psychological trauma related to the broadly understood emotional abandonment by the mother (Józefik, 1999; Williams, 1997).

Psychological mechanisms dominated by perfectionism and strong control result from a specific (described in psychoanalytical theories) emotional and cognitive "no entry system" for receiving and experiencing external stimuli. It is formed as a result of psychological trauma experienced during the preverbal period. The pattern of rejection and emotional coldness of the mother (or other primary caregiver) in relation to the infant shapes the early childhood system of psychological mechanisms of "closure" to emotional experience and all stimuli, which Gianna Williams (1997) termed the *"no entry system."* Bodily wasting and the anorexic restriction symptoms would be related, among others, to the above psychological background. Such patients require a more careful psychological diagnosis and a longer therapeutic contact to recognize the presence of early childhood (unconscious) preverbal traumas in relation to the maternal object. It seems that women with such a history might not have been included in the group of respondents covered by the diagnosis. Women with restrictive anorexia and experiencing this type of trauma may be recruited from among those with a low BMI and bodily wasting, which would lead them to seek hospitalization. Their level of wasting would make it impossible to conduct research for ethical reasons.

Analyzing the results of this study and referring them to the literature, it is worth pointing to certain similarities. They mainly concern the frequent occurrence of relational trauma (mental, physical, and sexual abuse) among patients with bulimia and bulimic anorexia (Kent et al., 1999; Kent & Waller, 2000; Monteleone et al., 2021; Vanderlinden & Palmisano, 2018; Wonderlich et al., 2001). The studies by Keel et al. (2001, 2010) are also significant in the area of impulsivity in bulimia and the presence of psychological trauma. On the other hand, the importance of relational trauma and traumatic events (emotional abandonment and deprivation of the sense of security during childhood) has been emphasized in studies on patients with eating disorders in various countries (Caslini et al., 2016; Collins et al., 2014; Franzoni et al., 2013; Hewett, 2015; Litwack et al., 2014; Madowitz et al., 2015; McCormack et al., 2014; Moulton et al., 2015; Racine & Wildes, 2015; Tahilani, 2015; Tasca et al., 2013). In Polish studies, the topic of trauma in eating disorders is very poorly explored (Izydorczyk, 2017a).

The role of traumatic events, and especially relational traumas, in eating disorders should be taken into account as an important indicator in psychological diagnosis and psychotherapy for this group of patients. While the relationship between traumatic experiences and the psychological readiness for compulsive behaviors and bulimic symptoms is complex and involves other mediating factors (e.g., alexithymia, dissociation, borderline personality disorder), taking into account the role of trauma in the diagnosis and treatment of patients with eating disorders is warranted and deserves further study.

Summarizing the above considerations, it bears emphasizing that if a young person seeks specialist help (from a doctor, psychologist, psychotherapist, or school counselor) because of personal difficulties, he bring with him his history, emotional experiences, psychological traumas, family relations (conflicts and communication patterns), patterns of attachment, and intergenerational messages and myths about food and nutrition.

References

Caslini, M., Bartoli, F, Crocamo, C., Dakanalis, A., Clerici, M., & Carra, G. (2016). Disentangling the association between child abuse and eating disorders: A systematic review and meta-analysis. *Psychosomatic Medicine*, 78(1), 79–90. 10.1097/PSY.0000000000000233

Collins, B., Fischer, S., Stojek, M., & Becker, K. (2014). The relationship of thought suppression and recent rape to disordered eating in emerging adulthood. *Journal of Adolescence, 37*(2), 113–121. 10.1016/j.adolescence.2013.11.002

Fonagy, P., Gergely, G., & Target, M. (2007). The parent-infant dyad and the construction of the subjective self. *Journal of Child Psychology and Psychiatry and Allied Disciplines, 48*(3–4), 288–328.

Fonagy, P., Luyten, P., & Bateman, A. (2015). Translation: Mentalizing as treatment target in borderline personality disorder. *Personality Disorders: Theory, Research, and Treatment, 6*(4), 380–392. 10.1037/per0000113

Fonagy, P., Luyten, P., Bateman, A., Gergely, G., Strathearn, L., Target, M., & Allison, E. (2013). Przywiązanie a patologia osobowości [Attachment and personality pathology]. In J. F. Clarkin, P. Fonagy, & G. O. Gabbard (Eds.), *Psychoterapia psychodynamiczna zaburzeń osobowości* [Psychodynamic psychotherapy of personality disorders] (pp. 61–119). Wydawnictwo Uniwersystetu Jagiellońskiego.

Franzoni, E., Gualandi, S., Caretti, V., Schimmenti, A., Di Pietro, E., Pellegrini, Craparo, G., Franchi, A., Verrotti, A., & Pellicciari, A. (2013). The relationship between alexithymia, shame, trauma, and body image disorders: Investigation over a large clinical sample. *Neuropsychiatric Disease and Treatment, 9*, 185–193. 10.2147/NDT.S34822

Garner, D. M. (2004). *EDI-3. Eating disorders inventory. Professional manual.* Psychological Assessment Resources, Inc.

Glickauf-Hughes, C., & Wells, M. (1997). *Object relations psychotherapy. An individual and integreative approach to diagnosis and treatment.* Jason Aronson, Inc.

Greenspan, S. I. (2000). *Rozwój umysłu. Emocjonalne podstawy inteligencji* [The growth of the mind]. Dom Wydawniczy Rebis.

Hartt, J., & Waller, G. (2002). Child abuse, dissociation and core beliefs in bulimic disorders. *Child Abuse & Neglect, 26*(9), 923–938. 10.1016/S0145-2134(02)00362-9

Hewett, J. (2015). *The impact of trauma and attachment on eating disorder symptomology.* [Doctoral dissertation, Loma Linda University]. Scholars Repository. https://scholarsrepository.llu.edu/etd/210/

Izydorczyk, B. (2015a). *Postawy i zachowania wobec własnego ciała w zaburzeniach odżywiania* [*Attitudes and behaviors towards the body in eating disorders*]. PWN.

Izydorczyk, B. (2015b). Psychological typology of females diagnosed with anorexia nervosa, bulimia nervosa or binge eating disorder. *Health Psychology Report, 3*(4), 312–325.

Izydorczyk B. (2017a). Trauma in relation to psychological characteristics in women with eating disorders. *Current Issues in Personality Psychology, 5*(4), 244–259. 10.5114/cipp.2017.67047

Izydorczyk, B. (2017b). Psychoterapia zaburzeń obrazu ciała w anoreksji i bulimii psychicznej: podejście integracyjne (zastosowanie terapii psychodynamicznej i technik psychodramy) [Psychotherapy of body image distortions in anorexia and bulimia: An integrative approach (using elements of psychodynamic psychotherapy and psychodrama techniques)]. *Psychoterapia,1* (180), 5–22.

Józefik, B. (Ed.) (1999). *Anoreksja i bulimia psychiczna. Rozumienie i leczenie zaburzeń odżywiania się* [*Anorexia and bulimia. Understanding and treatment of eating disorders*]. Wydawnictwo Uniwersytetu Jagiellońskiego.

Józefik, B. (2008). Koncepcja przywiązania a zaburzenia odżywiania – teoria i empiria [Attachment and eating disorders – theory and empirical results]. *Psychiatria Polska, 42*(2), 157–166.

Józefik, B., Iniewicz, G., & Ulasińska, R. (2010). Wzory przywiązania, samoocena i płeć psychologiczna w anoreksji i bulimii psychicznej [Attachment patterns, self-esteem, and psychological gender in anorexia and bulimia]. *Psychiatria Polska*, *44*(5), 665–676.

Keel, P. K., Gravener, J. A., Joiner, T. E. & Haedt, A. A. (2010). Twenty-year follow-up of bulimia nervosa and related eating disorders not otherwise specified. *International Journal Eating Disorders*, *43*(6), 492–497. 10.1002/eat.20743

Keel, P. K., Mitchell, J. E., Davis, T. L., & Crow, S. J. (2001). Relationship between depression and body dissatisfaction in women diagnosed with bulimia nervosa. *International Journal Eating Disorders*, *30*(1), 48–56. 10.1002/eat.1053

Kent, A., & Waller, G. (2000). Childhood emotional abuse and eating psycho-pathology. *Clinical Psychology Review*, *20*(7), 887–903. 10.1016/S0272-7358(99)00018-5

Kent, A., Waller, G., & Dagnan, D. A. (1999). A greater role of emotional than physical or sexual abuse in predicting disordered eating attitudes: The role of mediating variables. *International Journal of Eating Disorders*, *25*(2), 159–167. 10.1002/(SICI)1098-108X(199903)25:2%3C159::AID-EAT5%3E3.0.CO;2-F

Kubiak, A., & Sakson-Obada, O. (2016). Nawykowe samouszkodzenia a Ja cielesne [Repetetive self-injury and the body self]. *Psychiatria Polska*, *50*(1), 43–54. 10.12740/PP/44453

Krueger, D. W. (2002a). Psychodynamic perspective on body image. In T. F. Cash, & T. Pruzinsky (Eds.), *Body image. A handbook of theory, research, and clinical practice* (pp. 30–37). The Guilford Press.

Krueger, D. W. (2002b). *Integrating body self and psychological self. Creating a new story in psychoanalysis and psychotherapy*. Bruner-Routledge.

Krystal, H. (1977) Aspects of affect theory. *Bulletin of the Menninger Clinic*, *41*(1), 1–26.

Krystal, H. (1979). Alexithymia and psychotherapy. *The American Journal of Psychotherapy*, *33*(1), 17–31. 10.1176/appi.psychotherapy.1979.33.1.17

Krystal, H. (2000). *Trauma und Affekte – Posttraumtische Folgeerscheinungen und ihre Konsequenzen für die psychoanalytische Behandlungstechnik.* [*Paper presentation*]. Contemporary Psychoanalysis.

Litwack, S. D., Mitchell, K. R., Sloan, D. M., Reardon, A. F., & Miller, M. W. (2014). Eating disorder symptoms and comorbid psychopathology among male and female veterans. *General Hospital Psychiatry*, *36*(4), 406–410. 10.1016/j.genhosppsych.2014.03.013

Luban-Plozza, B., Poldinger, W., Kroger, F., & Wasilewski, B. (1995). *Zaburzenia psychosomatycznew praktyce lekarskiej* [*Psychosomatic disorders in medical practice*]. PZWL.

Madowitz, J., Matheson, B. E., & Liang, J. (2015). The relationship between eating disorders and sexual trauma. *Eating and Weight Disorders*, *20*(3), 281–293. 10.1007/s40519-015-0195-y

McCormack, L., Lewis, V., & Wells, J. R. (2014). Early life loss and trauma: Eating disorder onset in a middle- aged male – a case study. *American Journal of Men's Health*, *8*(2), 121–136. 10.1177/1557988313496838

McDougall, J. (2014). *Teatr ciała. Psychoanalityczne podejście do chorób psychoso-matycznych* [*Theatre of the body: A psychoanalytic approach to psychosomatic illness*]. Oficyna Ingenium.

Monteleone, A. M., Tzischinsky, O., Cascino, G., Pellegrino, F., Ruzzi, V. & Latzer, Y. (2021). The connection between childhood maltreatment and eating disorder psychopathology: A network analysis study in people with bulimia nervosa and with binge eating. *Eating and Weight Disorders*. 10.1007/s40519-021-01169-6

Moulton, S. J., Newman, E., Power, K., Swanson, V., & Day, K. (2015). Childhood trauma and eating psychopathology: A mediating role for dissociation and emotion dysregulation? *Child Abuse & Neglect, 39*, 167–174. 10.1016/j.chiabu. 2014.07.003

Racine, S. E., & Wildes, J. E. (2015). Emotion dysregulation and anorexia nervosa: An exploration of the role of childhood abuse. *International Journal of Eating Disorders*, 48(1), 55–58. 10.1002/eat.22364

Rzeszutek, M. & Schier, K. (2008). Doświadczenie utraty własnego ciała a obraz własnego ciała u młodych dorosłych [Experience of body loss and body image among young adults]. *Psychologia - Etologia – Genetyka, 17*, 89–110.

Sakson-Obada, O. (2008). Rozwój Ja cielesnego w kontekście wczesnej relacji z opiekunem [Development of the body Ego in the context of the early relationship with a caregiver]. *Roczniki Psychologiczne, 11*(2), 27–44.

Sakson-Obada, O. (2009a). *Pamięć ciała. Ja cielesne w relacji przywiązania i w traumie* [The body's memory. The body Self in attachment relationships and trauma]. Wydawnictwo Difin.

Sakson-Obada, O. (2009b). Trauma jako czynnik ryzyka dla zaburzeń Ja cielesnego [trauma as a risk factor for the disorders of the bodily ego]. *Przegląd Psychologiczny, 52*(3), 309–326.

Schier, K. (2020). *Samotne ciało* [The lonely body]. Wydawnictwo Scholar.

Skrzypska, N., & Suchańska, A. (2011). Uraz seksualny jako czynnik ryzyka zaburzeń doświadczania własnej cielesności [Sexual trauma as a risk factor of disorders in experiencing of one's own body]. *Seksuologia Polska, 9*(2), 51–56.

Tahilani, K. (2015). *Impact of self-efficacy and emotion dysregulation as mediators between trauma history and disordered eating* [Doctoral Dissertation, St. John's University]. ProQuest. https://search.proquest.com/dissertations-theses/impact-self-efficacy-emotion-dysregulation-as/docview/1586062351/se-2?accountid=14887

Tasca, G., Ritchie, K., Zachariades, F., Trinneer, A., Balfour, L., Demidenko, N., & Bissada, H. (2013). Attachment insecurity mediates the relationship between childhood trauma and eating disorder psychopathology in a clinical sample: A structural equation model. *Child Abuse & Neglect, 37*(11), 926–933. 10.1016/j.chiabu. 2013.03.004

Vanderlinden, J., & Palmisano, G. L. (2018). Trauma and the eating disorders: The state of the art. In A. Seubert & P. Virdi (Eds.), *Trauma-informed approaches to eating disorders* (pp. 13–30). Springer.

Williams, G. (1997). *Eating disorders and other pathologies. Internal landscapes and foreign bodies*. Taylor & Francis Group.

Wonderlich, S. A., Crosby, R. D., Mitchell, J. E., Thompson, K. M., Redlin, J., Demuth, G., Smyth, J., & Haseltine, B. (2001). Eating disturbance and sexual trauma in childhood and adulthood. *International Journal of Eating Disorders, 30*(4), 401–412. 10.1002/eat.1101

Żechowski, C. (2008). Polska wersja Kwestionariusza Zaburzeń Odżywiania (EDI) – adaptacja i normalizacja [Polish Version of Eating Disorder Inventory – adaptation and normalization]. *Psychiatria Polska, 42*(2), 179–193.

4 Psychological characteristics of patients with eating disorders

In contrast to the characteristics of the mechanisms of development of eating disorder symptoms commonly reported in medical literature, the definitions and psychological mechanisms of the so-called anorexic readiness and bigorexia are researched and discussed less frequently. Both these psychological states are related to distortions in body image and simultaneously to specific eating behaviors. Chapter 4 also presents the results of research describing the psychological characteristics of the three profiles – restrictive, bulimic, and youth – along with their levels of pressure and the internalization of sociocultural standards of body image present in social media.

Anorexic readiness and bigorexia: psychological characteristics

Anorexic readiness and bigorexia are two specific psychological phenomena that are very closely related to body image distortions and the use of specific eating behaviors to obtain an idealized body image. The anorexic readiness syndrome can be placed between specific and nonspecific eating disorders (Ziółkowska, 2000, 2001). Contrary to nonspecific eating disorders, its etiology is conditioned by personality factors, harmful relationships, susceptibility to cultural influences, as well as specific symptoms (Ziółkowska, 2000, 2001). The anorexic readiness syndrome is conditioned by numerous social and cultural factors. Research on the anorexic readiness syndrome increasingly often focuses on sociocultural pressure and the role of mass media in creating the ideal of female body image, which, in turn, influences its internalization and perceived dissatisfaction with one's own body among adolescent girls (Brytek-Matera & Rybicka-Klimczyk, 2012; Izydorczyk & Gut, 2018).

In turn, bigorexia, or muscle dysmorphia, is most often defined as an excessive, abnormal preoccupation with and concern for one's muscle mass and its growth while maintaining a constant low level of body fat (Michalska et al., 2016; Morgan, 2000). Pope et al. (1993) called bigorexia symptoms "reverse anorexia," emphasizing their differences and similarities. The differences include the goal of bigorexic behaviors (to increase muscle

DOI: 10.4324/9781003251088-4

mass and body weight). On the other hand, the similarities concern a distorted and unsatisfying body image, which results in behaviors aimed at reducing body fat despite a healthy body mass index (BMI; Michalska et al., 2016). Pope et al. (2002) define bigorexia as the "Adonis complex," pointing to the importance of social determinants of the ideal male body image. The Adonis complex includes behaviors that result from a distorted body image and the related need to conform to sociocultural body image standards (Eynon & Lowry, 2013). The ICD-10 introduced the category of dysmorphophobia (nondelusional), including it within hypochondriac disorders. The DSM-V introduced the category of "muscle dysmorphia," including it among dysmorphic body disorders within obsessive–compulsive disorders.

Due to the increasing tendency to develop both anorexic readiness and bigorexia, it is worth taking into account the measurement of both these types of behavior in the process of psychological diagnosis. This may be an important element of preparing patients for psychological therapy.

Anorexic readiness: diagnostic indicators

The anorexic readiness syndrome is a theoretical construct comprising a set of behaviors, thoughts, and feelings that may be a potential source of abnormal (anorexic) eating behaviors and perception of own body image (Ziółkowska, 2001). It includes a spectrum of indicators that determine the risk of developing anorexia or other eating disorders (Ziółkowska, 2001). These include, but are not limited to:

- a strong need for control and perfectionist behaviors only in selected areas of activity (as opposed to anorexia, where trait perfectionism is high, manifests itself in many areas of life, and can take an obsessive–compulsive form);
- increased interest in food and its nutritional value;
- increased interest in diets and/or weight control methods;
- periodically increasing physical activity;
- susceptibility to the influence of mass media (especially visual media);
- excessive focus on the body and appearance;
- underestimating own attractiveness and comparisons with idealized body image standards;
- emotional lability mainly determined by the attitude toward food and the body;
- a tendency to control body weight and size, which may be accompanied by emotional stress;
- an increased need for competition and/or increased perfectionism and/or emotional lability.

Połom (2015) distinguished three categories of anorexic behaviors. The first includes behaviors based on weight reduction and appearance control (preoccupation with the caloric value of consumed food, controlling food and eating, body size, and weight, and intensive physical activity). The second category includes behaviors related to excessive concentration on own appearance, overestimation of own body size, exaggerated care for appearance, and constant comparisons with the ideal female body image promoted in media (Korolik & Kochan-Wójcik, 2015; Połom, 2015). The third category includes personality traits such as perfectionism and the need for achievement and constant control (Izydorczyk, 2015a, 2015b; Józefik, 2014; Mikołajczyk & Samochowiec, 2004a, 2004b). They are often strengthened by the family environment, which, by placing high demands on the child, pressures them to strive toward perfection and stimulates competition (Połom, 2015). Additionally, when analyzing anorexic behaviors, it is worth taking into account their emotional dimension, namely, the associated emotional lability and tension related to body image and weight (Ziółkowska, 2001). Adolescent girls are at particular risk for developing the anorexic readiness syndrome (Józefik, 1999; Ziółkowska, 2001). Anorexic readiness includes a spectrum of symptoms related to body image distortions in which there is a large discrepancy between the need to have the idealized body image and the negative assessment of own actual appearance. This discrepancy becomes a source of excessively restrictive or impulsive behaviors toward eating and physical activity in order to cause weight loss and/or to obtain the idealized muscle mass. It is often stimulated by the internalization of sociocultural standards of an excessively thin or muscular figure (Brytek-Matera & Rybicka-Klimczyk, 2012).

Scientific research increasingly often refers to anorexic readiness or the sociocultural syndrome of willingness to restrict eating (Izydorczyk & Gut, 2018; Ziółkowska, 2001). Young women presenting risky (excessively restrictive and/or bulimic) eating behaviors tend to overestimate the importance of external appearance (Ziółkowska, 2001). In case of anorexic readiness, it is difficult to distinguish a regular diet from destructive behaviors (Chytra-Gędek & Kobierecka, 2008). Similarly, patients exhibiting anorexic readiness usually have normal body weight, but they might show a tendency toward comparisons with models in the media. They also experience difficulties in building emotional relationships in the family system – most often the contact between the caregivers and the child is/was either too close or too distant. In families of patients with eating disorders, family relations and roles are characterized by involvement in marital problems, excessive control, need deprivation, distorted boundaries due to overprotective attitudes, and so forth.

When differentiating between patients with the anorexic readiness syndrome and patients with anorexia regarding the influence of sociocultural factors, it is worth considering that the former are selectively susceptible to the influence of mass media on comparisons of their body image to the promoted standards of attractiveness. On the other hand, patients with anorexia additionally engage in numerous compulsive behaviors, striving to obtain an appearance identical to the culturally promoted ideal (Ziółkowska, 2001). Moreover, the anorexic readiness syndrome is characterized by a tendency toward food restrictions (Chytra-Gędek & Kobierecka, 2008; Ziółkowska, 2001). It is conditioned by many factors, for example, environmental and subjective ones. The first group includes upbringing style and family relations (Ziółkowska, 2000, 2001). In families with a large emotional distance between the members, where professional/educational success is valued the most, the child may feel lonely, insecure, and deprived of self-worth, which favors the development of anti-health behaviors (Ziółkowska, 2001). Additionally, abnormalities appear in families where high expectations are placed on the child, including expectations regarding his body shape. According to Goodsitt (see Ziółkowska & Wycisk, 2010), a perfectionist and controlling upbringing style plays a key role in the etiology of eating disorders. According to the study by Połom (2015), family pressure and seeking of parental acceptance have a large impact on achievement motivation among girls. Połom points out that in families focused on strengthening their daughters' achievement motivation and perfectionism in many areas of everyday functioning, girls may develop anorexic behaviors in the future.

Anorexic readiness is most evident in the extremely positive affirmation of a thin figure, in which thinness is equated with popularity and broadly conceptualized life success. According to Chytra-Gędek and Kobierecka (2008), these beliefs are influenced by the cultural and media norm of thinness. Similar conclusions can be drawn from the study by Owsiejczyk (2007), which showed that most of the surveyed women believed a thin figure and attractive appearance to be sources of happiness and success.

The subjective predictors of the anorexic readiness syndrome and eating disorders include low self-esteem, extreme perfectionism (Korolik & Kochan-Wójcik, 2015; Ziółkowska, 2001), and strong achievement motivation (Józefik, 1999). This is referred to in the literature as extrinsic motivation (Ziółkowska, 2001). It concerns both the environmental pressure of the individual, in which peers play an important role, as well as the broader cultural pressure.

An additional, important factor that may directly influence abnormal behaviors and attitudes related to eating is the style of coping with difficult situations (Ziółkowska, 2001). Among girls at risk for anorexia, the most frequently used coping strategy is emotion-focused coping, where anorexic behaviors serve to reduce emotional tension (Jaros, 2014). Emotion-focused coping in conjunction with stressors may contribute to the development of anorexic readiness. Stressors may include difficult family and school situations as well as sociocultural influences. However, in addition to anorexic readiness, it is also worth considering orthorexia and differentiating it from anorexic readiness.

Orthorexia: diagnostic indicators

Orthorexia is a "pathological fixation on eating the right and healthy food" (Stochel et al., 2015). Research on orthorexia has been conducted by

Loreznzo Maria Donini and his team in Italy (qtd. in Stochel et al., 2015). However, a tool for measuring orthorexia indicators called ORTO-15 has also been developed in Poland (Stochel et al., 2015). The following criteria of orthorexia are distinguished:

- the tendency to choose or avoid specific foods, linked with health concerns;
- choosing foods according to their quality, not their quantity or caloric value (which is important in anorexic behaviors);
- motivation related to health concerns (in anorexic behaviors, motivation is related to weight loss or control);
- failure to follow diets, which causes anxiety and guilt – similar to anorexic behaviors (Janas-Kozik et al., 2012);
- elements of obsessive thinking about food, showing an impact on self-esteem and interpersonal relationships (especially in places where food considered "forbidden" by the patient is available, Dittfeld et al., 2013).

Apart from anorexic readiness and orthorexia, bigorexia is also emerging in the literature as a new type of eating disorder. The psychological characteristics and diagnostic criteria of bigorexia indicate the central role of body image (especially the desire to have a muscle mass corresponding to sociocultural standards) in driving bigorexic behavior. The psychological diagnosis of body image may be important for measuring the severity of the tendency toward harmful bigorexic behaviors, provoked by body image distortions in the area of muscle mass and internalized esthetic standards.

Bigorexia: diagnostic indicators

Bigorexia predominantly affects men, but occasionally also women (Chung, 2001). It usually appears around the age of 19, meaning that it includes both adults as well as adolescents (Olivardia, 2001). A review of research shows a higher frequency of bigorexia in bodybuilders (Babusa & Túry, 2011; Guerra-Torres & Arango-Vélez, 2015), professional soldiers (Campagna & Bowsher, 2016), and personal fitness trainers (Diehl & Baghurst, 2016). Studies also indicate numerous determinants of bigorexia – from biological to psychological and sociocultural factors (Leit et al., 2002). For example, Olivardia (2001) lists body weight as a biological determinant, self-esteem as a psychological one, and the influence of mass media messages (e.g., "having a muscular body is the basis of masculinity") as a sociocultural one. In turn, describing the determinants of bigorexic behavior, Grieve (2007) emphasizes the importance of body dissatisfaction stimulated by sociocultural pressure as a significant factor intensifying bigorexia symptoms. Among the psychological determinants of bigorexia, he also lists perfectionism and the drive for thinness (Grieve, 2007).

The DSM-V (American Psychiatric Association, 2013) indicates the following diagnostic criteria for bigorexia (muscle dysmorphia):

- preoccupation with one or more imaginary body defects;
- exhibiting certain behaviors or thoughts in response to feelings of dissatisfaction with own appearance (e.g., looking in a mirror, comparing themselves to others);
- dissatisfaction with own appearance causes significant deterioration in well-being and social, professional, or other spheres of life;
- preoccupation with appearance cannot be better explained by other mental disorders (such as eating disorders).

Psychological diagnosis of bigorexic behaviors should include the DSM-V criteria as well as a description of behaviors and thoughts focused around dissatisfaction with the body and muscle mass. These lead to excessive guilt due to these perceived deficiencies, which cannot be explained by other mental disorders (e.g., bulimia or anorexia). Bigorexia may also co-occur with obsessive–compulsive disorders and affective disorders (including depression and bipolar disorder, Olivardia, 2001).

When diagnosing bigorexia, it is worth paying attention to the following behaviors:

- limiting and avoiding undressing in public places (regardless of muscle mass) due to the accompanying discomfort, anxiety, and fear;
- intensive physical exercises which might lead to injuries, using diets and physical exercise despite significant deterioration in physical and/or mental well-being;
- subordinating the daily schedule to physical exercise (strict adherence to the exercise schedule due to persistent thoughts about muscle mass, repeatedly looking in the mirror or other reflective surfaces in public, etc.);
- constant comparisons of own body shape with people from your immediate surroundings;
- daily weighing and measuring of muscle circumference to detect muscle gain;
- limiting activities that interfere with physical exercise (addiction to exercise), leading to a deterioration in family, social, and professional functioning;
- using substances stimulating muscle growth;
- engaging in physical exercises characterized by high intensity and duration, ignoring physical discomfort or pain caused by the exercises;
- constant focus on improving exercise and muscle mass, which also limits other social and personal activity, for example, causing sexual dysfunction (Mangweth et al., 2001; Pope et al., 2000). Patients with bigorexia also use various dietary supplements and substances (including

hormonal agents) to achieve the desired body musculature (Hernández-Martínez et al., 2017; Zięba et al., 2018).

Theories of bigorexic behavior include the following:

- Biopsychosocial: explaining the biological, psychological, and cultural basis of bigorexia by reference to low self-esteem combined with the sociocultural pressure to achieve the ideal body image (Leit et al., 2002; Olivardia, 2001; Pope et al., 1997).
- Grieve's model (2007), which identifies important factors in the etiology of bigorexia (socioenvironmental, emotional, psychological, and physiological), including dissatisfaction with body image and overstimulation with ideal body image norms promoted in the media.

Psychological profiles of patients with eating disorders

Psychological theories indicate the importance of assessing the profile of psychological and personality traits in the diagnosis and treatment of eating disorders (Mikołajczyk & Samochowiec, 2004a, 2004b). On the other hand, clinical practice confirms such profile assessment is performed only rarely. Meanwhile, it should be noted that the psychological diagnosis of personality is related to the specific functioning of not only the mental Self, but also the body Self (Izydorczyk, 2011, 2017; Krueger, 2002a). Identifying the specific features and development level of the patient's personality structure (thus, the body image distortions and the development level of the body Self) may constitute – apart from the medical diagnostic criteria – important elements supporting treatment, especially psychotherapy. For this reason, according to evidence-based practice, such profile assessment should be complementary to psychotherapy of patients with eating disorders. It is indicated in the literature (Garner, 2004; Izydorczyk, 2013a, 2013b, 2015b, 2017; Mikołajczyk & Samochowiec, 2004a, 2004b) that the clinical diagnosis of eating disorders should take into account the assessment of the psychological features presented below.

Garner (2004) lists the following psychological features which may be helpful in diagnosing the psychological profile of patients with eating disorders:

- low self-esteem (an important predictor of eating disorders);
- body image distortions – especially centered around the discrepancy between the real body image, the BMI, and the internalized perfect body image;
- negative body esteem (dissatisfaction with the body manifested both in thoughts and emotional experiences);
- perfectionism (especially in patients with anorexic readiness and anorexia);

- impulsivity (especially in patients with bulimia and binge eating disorder);
- deficits in interoceptive awareness (disturbances in the perception of physiological stimuli, for example, pain, hunger, satiety);
- tendencies toward so-called "bulimic thinking" (excessive concern with eating, overeating, and purging due to associating eating with anxiety, together with a constant, strong emotional tension and the fear of gaining weight);
- fear of gaining weight (fat phobia – important in specific types of eating disorders);
- fear of taking on adult social roles (especially in adolescents and young adults, related to the sphere of interpersonal relationships);
- insecurity and distrust in interpersonal relationships – fear of building lasting emotional bonds with other people.

The basic psychological profile of patients with specific eating disorders (especially anorexia, bulimia, as well as binge eating disorder) allows for making the first diagnostic hypotheses about the patient's functioning through the process of building the therapeutic alliance and relationship early in the treatment. However, apart from the psychological profile, clinical diagnosis of patients with eating disorders for the purpose of psychotherapy should also include indicators of the sociocultural influence on body image and BMI. The tools for measuring cognitions related to body image (internalized schema, bodily boundaries, perception of and thoughts about the body) include projective tests recognized in this area, which are mainly drawing methods, for example, drawing a body image and the Thompson Figure Test (Thompson & Altabe, 1991). The body dissatisfaction subscale in Garner's *Eating Disorders Questionnaire* (Garner, 2004) can be used to assess the level of negative emotions related to the body. This questionnaire also allows for assessing affective control (perfectionism, maturity fears, bulimic tendencies, drive for thinness), interpersonal distrust (difficulties in building emotional connections with others), as well as ineffectiveness (low self-esteem and a sense of worthlessness).

The *Questionnaire of Sociocultural Attitudes to Physical Appearance* by Thompson, in the Polish adaptation of Izydorczyk and Lizińczyk (2020) can be used to measure the intensity and nature of self-destructive behaviors related to the body and eating. Considering the comprehensive measurement of psychological and sociocultural variables, it is worth expanding the psychological diagnosis by describing the so-called specific psychological types of patients with eating disorders. Such types represent different patterns of body image distortions as well as psychological and sociocultural influences. The research conducted by Izydorczyk and her team in 2015–2018 identified three such types in a sample of 121 girls and young women with anorexia, bulimia, and binge eating disorder. The clinical characteristics of the identified types are presented below.

Psychological types among girls and young women with eating disorders: own research

The ICD-10 (World Health Organization, 1993) and DSM-V (American Psychiatric Association, 2013) diagnoses of eating disorders are mainly based on symptom criteria (mainly behavioral), disregarding the psychological features and body image distortions. A *K*-means cluster analysis was used for the psychometric and clinical diagnosis of group differences in a sample of 121 young Polish women. It was checked whether the differences between the surveyed women and girls with diagnoses of different eating disorders, verified at an earlier stage, would be reflected in the cluster analysis. The distribution of the selected clusters (psychological types) and eating disorders diagnoses they contained was analyzed together with the distribution of psychological and sociocultural features related to body image. It was examined whether the distinguished clusters would contain only homogeneous diagnoses of restrictive anorexia, bulimia nervosa, and binge eating disorder or whether the clusters would be heterogeneous, that is, would combine different diagnoses. The *K*-means cluster analysis was used to group the participants into relatively homogeneous classes based on the similarity on the independent variable scores, expressed by the similarity function. Such data analysis methods find particular application in various medical fields (grouping diseases, symptoms, or treatments to develop an effective and reliable classification and to assist in psychological therapy; Hartigan & Wong, 1979). Data from medical records containing a description of the psychodynamic diagnostic indicators of the participants' personality structure were also used to diagnose their profiles.

The cluster analysis identified three clusters in the sample with statistically significant differences in terms of BMI, the measured psychological traits, and body image variables (see Fig. 4.1; Tables 4.1–4.3).

Due to the demonstrated specificity of each cluster in terms of the measured psychological and sociocultural factors, the following psychological types were proposed: restrictive (Cluster 1), impulsive (Cluster 2), and adolescent girls (Cluster 3).

Restrictive type (Cluster 1): psychological profile, diagnostic indicators, and psychological therapy recommendations

Cluster 1, termed the restrictive type, comprised 52 women with a mean age of 21 (the median and mean were similar), mean body weight of 53 kg, and mean BMI of 18.59 (borderline underweight). In this cluster, significant intergroup variation in BMI was observed (e.g., the highest reported BMI in this cluster was 26).

Women representing the restrictive type showed the highest body dissatisfaction (suggesting a high level of negative emotions associated with

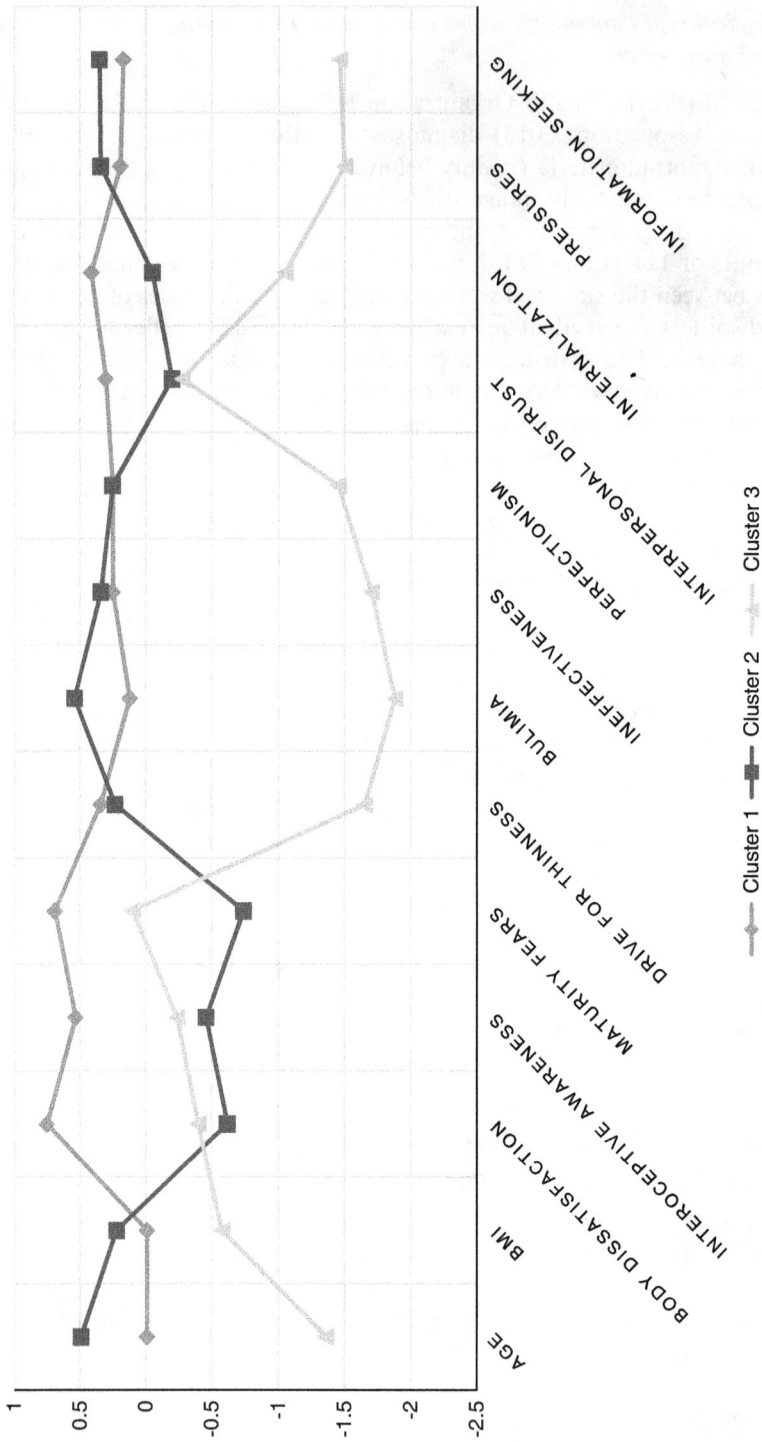

Figure 4.1 Characteristics of clusters of girls and young women with eating disorders (*N* = 121) in terms of mean age, BMI, psychological traits, body dissatisfaction, and sociocultural factors related to body image.

Table 4.1 Age, BMI, psychological and sociocultural variables, and body dissatisfaction in the sample of girls and young women with eating disorders (N = 121). ANOVA, Fisher's test

Variable	Cluster 1 (N = 52)	Cluster 2 (N = 51)	Cluster 3 (N = 18)	df	F	p
Age	−0.01	0.49	−1.36	118	36.11	.001
BMI	−0.01	0.22	−0.58	118	4.45	.014
Body dissatisfaction	0.75	−0.62	−0.40	118	44.37	.001
Interoceptive awareness	0.53	−0.46	−0.24	118	16.84	.001
Maturity fears	0.69	−0.74	0.10	118	46.54	.001
Drive for thinness	0.34	0.23	−1.65	118	55.25	.001
Bulimia	0.12	0.54	−1.88	118	115.06	.001
Ineffectiveness	0.25	0.34	−1.70	118	61.03	.001
Perfectionism	0.25	0.25	−1.45	118	34.59	.001
Interpersonal distrust	0.30	−0.20	−0.28	118	4.24	.017
Internalizations	0.41	−0.05	−1.05	118	18.37	.001
Pressures	0.19	0.34	−1.50	118	39.70	.001
Information-seeking	0.17	0.35	−1.46	118	36.68	.001

Table 4.2 Mean age, BMI, and psychological and sociocultural factors in Cluster 1 – restrictive type (N = 52)

Variables	M	Me	Min	Max	SD
Age	21.15	21.00	14.00	29.0	3.96
Weight	53.54	53.00	30.10	115.0	12.92
BMI	18.59	18.50	13.60	26.0	2.98
Body dissatisfaction	26.58	25.50	11.00	40.0	8.23
Interoceptive awareness	18.69	19.50	6.00	28.0	5.35
Maturity fears	16.96	17.00	5.00	27.0	5.07
Drive for thinness	19.15	18.50	15.00	27.0	2.48
Bulimia	15.69	18.00	1.00	21.0	4.83
Ineffectiveness	17.19	17.00	11.00	22.0	2.14
Perfectionism	16.02	16.00	6.00	28.0	3.52
Interpersonal distrust	19.13	18.00	13.00	30.0	3.49
Internalization	25.90	26.00	14.00	38.0	4.17
Pressures	22.46	23.50	7.00	32.0	4.53
Information seeking	25.44	27.00	7.00	36.0	7.98

Note: M = mean, Me = median, SD = standard deviation.

body image), high drive for thinness (indicating significantly more frequent restrictive eating behaviors compared to other clusters), the highest interoceptive awareness deficits among all clusters, high ineffectiveness, and relatively low bulimic tendencies. Cluster 1 also included women with the highest level of perfectionism, interpersonal distrust, and internalization of sociocultural body image standards (see Table 4.1). Women in Cluster 1 also had different eating disorder diagnoses (anorexia: 50%; bulimia: 40%; binge

Table 4.3 Mean age, BMI, and psychological and sociocultural factors in Cluster 2 – bulimic type (N = 51)

Variable	M	Me	Min	Max	SD
Age	23.33	24.00	18.00	29.00	3.223
Weight	52.63	52.00	37.00	75.00	6.931
BMI	19.44	19.33	12.00	44.92	4.494
Body dissatisfaction	13.59	14.00	0.00	29.00	6.664
Interoceptive awareness	12.25	13.00	0.00	24.00	6.575
Maturity fears	7.65	7.00	0.00	15.00	4.660
Drive for thinness	18.67	19.00	15.00	20.00	1.178
Bulimia	18.47	19.00	10.00	21.00	2.788
Ineffectiveness	17.55	17.00	10.00	21.00	2.595
Perfectionism	16.02	16.00	10.00	29.00	2.731
Interpersonal distrust	17.49	18.00	12.00	20.00	1.433
Internalization	23.61	24.00	11.00	29.00	3.595
Pressures	23.27	24.00	12.00	29.00	4.119
Information-seeking	26.88	27.00	18.00	37.00	4.714

Note: M = mean, Me = Median, SD = standard deviation.

eating disorder : 10%). Data from clinical interviews and medical records indicated that apart from the medical diagnoses, women in Cluster 1 had a psychodynamic diagnosis of the neurotic personality structure. They exhibited anxious (10% of the sample) and obsessive–compulsive (30% of the sample) personality traits. Cluster 1 was small, which means that the current results and conclusions should be interpreted with caution. However, from the clinical perspective, it seems significant that this cluster mainly comprised young women characterized by restrictive, obsessive–compulsive mechanisms of emotional regulation.

Bulimic type (Cluster 2): psychological profile, diagnostic indicators, and psychological therapy recommendations

Cluster 2, termed the bulimic type, comprised 51 women with a mean age of 23.33 (the median and mean were similar) mean weight of 52.63 kg, and mean and BMI of 19.44 (within norm). Women in Cluster 2 showed the highest intensity of bulimic tendencies in the total sample (slightly higher than Cluster 1 and significantly higher than Cluster 3) as well as the highest ineffectiveness (see Tables 4.1–4.3).

Women in Cluster 2 (bulimic type), similarly to Cluster 1 (restrictive type) experienced a very high degree of pressures and internalization of sociocultural body image standards. They also reported the highest frequency of seeking body image information out of the total sample. Compared to other participants, women in Cluster 2 showed lower body dissatisfaction, interoceptive awareness deficits, and maturity fears (see Table 4.3).

Table 4.4 Mean age, BMI, and psychological and sociocultural factors in Cluster 3 –
adolescent type (N = 18)

Variable	M	Me	Min	Max	SD
Age	15.39	15.50	12.00	18.00	1.754
Weight	43.17	42.50	30.00	61.00	9.060
BMI	16.46	16.05	13.30	21.60	2.532
Body dissatisfaction	15.67	16.50	5.00	28.00	5.488
Interoceptive awareness	13.67	13.50	6.00	20.00	4.187
Maturity fears	13.11	12.00	6.00	22.00	5.132
Drive for thinness	10.50	8.50	1.00	21.00	6.784
Bulimia	2.33	1.00	0.00	10.00	3.678
Ineffectiveness	9.94	10.00	5.00	18.00	3.827
Perfectionism	8.61	7.00	3.00	21.00	5.031
Interpersonal distrust	17.22	18.50	9.00	28.00	5.429
Internalization	18.61	18.50	8.00	30.00	6.723
Pressures	12.89	13.00	6.00	23.00	4.825
Information-seeking	12.44	12.50	5.00	21.00	4.617

Note: M = mean, Me = Median, SD = standard deviation.

Cluster 2 women also displayed interpersonal distrust at a level similar to the youngest respondents (Cluster 3, adolescent type). This may mean that bulimic women have lower insecurity and distrust in relationships than women displaying the restrictive type of personality (Cluster 1).

In this cluster, perfectionism scores were similar to those of restrictive personality type women, but higher than those of adolescent girls. Drive for thinness was lower than for restrictive personality type women, but higher than for adolescent girls (see Tables 4.1–4.4). Bulimia predominated in the distribution of ICD-10 diagnoses in Cluster 2 (60%), with binge eating disorder (30%) and bulimic anorexia (10%) being less frequent. Data from clinical interviews and medical records indicated that, apart from medical diagnoses, women in Cluster 2 also had a psychodynamic diagnosis of the neurotic level of the personality structure (20%) with obsessive–compulsive or narcissistic personality traits (20%) and borderline personality structure (40%).

Adolescent type (Cluster 3): psychological profile, diagnostic indicators, and psychological therapy recommendations

Cluster 3, the adolescent type, was made up of 18 girls with a mean age of just over 15 years and mean BMI of 16.46 (below the underweight range). They were the youngest in the entire sample. Interestingly, this cluster comprised both girls with anorexia (40%), bulimia (40%), binge eating disorder, as well as purging and/or restrictive dieting (20%).

Women in Cluster 3 reported body dissatisfaction and interoceptive awareness deficits scores on a similar level to women with the bulimic personality type. On the other hand, maturity fears were similar between Clusters 1 and 3, and much higher than among the oldest women in Cluster 2. Of particular note is the fact that adolescent women reported the lowest average intensity of internalization and the pressure of sociocultural body image standards (see Table 4.4).

Young adult women with the restrictive and bulimic personality types showed similar levels of internalization of and pressures from sociocultural body image standards, which were much higher than among the teenage girls in the sample. This significant difference in the impact of sociocultural body image factors between adolescents and young adult women with the restrictive and bulimic personality types may have many causes: the specificity of the sample, the measures used in the study, BMI measurement, and the choice of measures for the psychological and sociocultural variables. However, from the perspective of developmental psychology and psychological theories (cognitive, psychoanalytical, and systems theory) explaining the psychopathology of eating disorders, the predictive importance of sociocultural factors for body image distortions in the period of early adulthood should be particularly highlighted (Izydorczyk & Sitnik-Warchulska, 2018).

According to Blos (qtd. in Schier, 1993) the adolescent girls in this study could be considered to have been in the developmental period termed "adolescence proper." This period is associated with many psychological processes, particularly those related to separation and individuation, that is, the formation of a complete (psychological, social, professional, sexual) identity and the crystallization of the structure of the Self. Separation and individuation may be more important than sociocultural factors alone in predicting body image distortions in adolescent girls aged 15 years with anorexia and bulimia. In this study, the BMI of adolescent girls presenting symptoms of anorexia or bulimia (Cluster 3, the adolescent personality type) most often presented with body wasting. Hence, it can be hypothesized that sociocultural influences on adolescents' body image may be modified by their psychophysical state and unconscious psychological processes.

References

American Psychiatric Association. (2013). *Diagnostic and statistical manual of mental disorders* (5th ed.). 10.1176/appi.books.9780890425596

Babusa, B., & Túry, F. (2011). Nosological classification and assessment of muscle dysmorphia. *Psychiatria Hungarica Journal, 26*(3), 158–166.

Brytek-Matera A., & Rybicka-Klimczyk A. (2012). Ocena nasilenia objawów syndromu gotowości anorektycznej u młodych kobiet – badania pilotażowe [Assessing anorexic readiness in young women – a pilot study]. *Studia Psychologica, 12*(2), 23–36.

Campagna, J., & Bowsher, B. (2016). Prevalence of body dysmorphic disorder and muscle dysmorphia among entry-level military personnel. *Military Medicine, 181*(5), 494–501. 10.7205/MILMED-D-15-00118

Chung, B. (2001). Muscle dysmorphia: A critical review of the proposed criteria. *Perspectives in Biology and Medicine*, *44*(4), 565–574. 10.1353/pbm.2001.0062

Chytra-Gędek, W., & Kobierecka, A. (2008). Gotowość anorektyczna u dziewcząt i młodych kobiet [Anorexic readiness among girls and young women], *Psychiatria*, *5*(1), 7–12.

Diehl, B., & Baghurst, T. (2016). Biopsychosocial factors in drives for muscularity and muscle dysmorphia among personal trainers. *Cogent Psychology*, *3*(1), 1–20. 10.1080/23311908.2016.1243194

Dittfeld, A., Koszowska, A., Fizia, K., & Ziora, K. (2013). *Ortoreksja – nowe zaburzenie odżywiania* [Orthorexia – a new eating disorder]. *Annales Academiae Medicae Silesiensis*, *67*(6), 393–399.

Eynon, M., & Lowry, R. (2013). Role of physical activity on the "Adonis complex." [Poster presentation]. British Psychological Society DHP Annual Conference. Brighton, England.

Garner, D. M. (2004). *EDI-3. Eating Disorders Inventory. Professional Manual*. Psychological Assessment Resources, Inc.

Grieve, F. (2007). A conceptual model of factors contributing to the development of muscle dysmorphia. *Eating Disorders*, *15*(1), 63–80. 10.1080/10640260601044535

Guerra-Torres, J., & Arango-Vélez, E. (2015). Muscle dysmorphia among competitive bodybuilders. *Revista Politécnica*, *11*(20), 39–48.

Hartigan J. A., & Wong M. A. (1979). A k-means clustering algorithm. *Journal of the Royal Statistical Society: Series C (Applied Statistics)*, *28*(1), 100–108. 10.2307/2346830

Hernández-Martínez, A., González-Martí, I., & Jordán, O. (2017). Detection of muscle dysmorphia symptoms in male weightlifters. *Anales de Psicología/Annals of Psychology*, *33*(1), 204–210. 10.6018/analesps.33.1.233311

Izydorczyk, B. (2011). A psychological profile of the bodily self characteristics in women suffering from bulimia nervosa. In P. Hay (Ed.), *New insights into the prevention and treatment of bulimia nervosa* (pp. 147–167). Intech Open Access Publisher.

Izydorczyk, B. (2013a). A psychological diagnosis of the structure of the body self in a group. *Archives of Psychiatry and Psychotherapy*, *13*(2), 21–30.

Izydorczyk, B. (2013b). Selected psychological traits and body image characteristics in females suffering from binge eating disorder. *Archives of Psychiatry and Psychotherapy*, *15*(1), 19–33.

Izydorczyk, B. (2015a). *Postawy i zachowania wobec własnego ciała w zaburzeniach odżywiania* [Attitudes and behaviors towards the body in eating disorders]. PWN.

Izydorczyk, B. (2015b). Psychological typology of females diagnosed with anorexia nervosa, bulimia nervosa or binge eating disorder. *Health Psychology Report*, *3*(4), 312–325.

Izydorczyk, B. (2017). Psychoterapia zaburzeń obrazu ciała w anoreksji i bulimii psychicznej: podejście integracyjne (zastosowanie terapii psychodynamicznej i technik psychodramy) [Psychotherapy of body image distortions in anorexia and bulimia: An integrative approach (using elements of psychodynamic psychotherapy and psychodrama techniques)]. *Psychoterapia*,*1*(180), 5–22.

Izydorczyk, B., & Gut, A. (2018). Samoocena i wpływ socjokulturowy na wizerunek ciała a gotowość do zachowań anorektycznych [Self-esteem and sociocultuar influenecs on body image and anorexic readiness]. *Czasopismo Psychologiczne*, *1*(24), 213–226.

Izydorczyk, B., & Lizińczyk, S. (2020). The Polish adaptation of the sociocultural attitudes towards appearance SATAQ 3 questionnaire. *Health Psychology Report*, *8*(1), 68–82. 10.5114/hpr.2020.91443

Izydorczyk, B., & Sitnik-Warchulska, K. (2018). Sociocultural appearance standards and risk factors for eating disorders in adolescents and women of various ages. *Frontiers in Psychology*, 9, 429, 1–21. 10.3389/fpsyg.2018.00429

Janas-Kozik, M., Zejda, J., Stochel, M., Brożek, G., Janas, A., & Jelonek, I. (2012). Ortoreksja – nowe rozpoznanie? [Orthorexia – a new diagnosis?]. *Psychiatria Polska*, *46*(3), 441–450.

Jaros, K. (2014). Style radzenia sobie ze stresem u dziewcząt z grupy ryzyka anoreksji [Styles of coping with stress among adolescent girls at risk for anorexia]. *Teraźniejszość – Człowiek – Edukacja*, *65*(1), 93–107.

Józefik, B. (Ed.) (1999). *Anoreksja i bulimia psychiczna. Rozumienie i leczenie zaburzeń odżywiania się [Anorexia and bulimia. Understanding and treatment of eating disorders]*. Wydawnictwo Uniwersytetu Jagiellońskiego.

Józefik, B. (2014). *Kultura, ciało, (nie)jedzenie* [Culture, body, (not)eating]. Wydawnictwo Uniwersytetu Jagiellońskiego.

Korolik, A., & Kochan-Wójcik, M. (2015). Anorexia readiness syndrome and sensitivity to body boundaries breaches. *Polish Journal of Applied Psychology*, *13*(4), 109–122.

Krueger, D. W. (2002a). Psychodynamic perspective on body image. In T. F. Cash, & T. Pruzinsky (Eds.), *Body image. A handbook of theory, research, and clinical practice* (pp. 30–37). The Guilford Press.

Leit, R., Gray, J., & Pope, H. (2002). The media's representation of the ideal male body: A cause for muscle dysmorphia? *International Journal of Eating Disorders*, *31*(3), 334–338. 10.1002/eat.10019

Mangweth, B., Pope, H., Kemmler, G., Ebenbichler, C., Hausmann, A., De Col, C., Kreutner, B., Kinzl, J., & Biebl, W. (2001). Body image and psychopathology in male bodybuilders. *Psychotherapy and Psychosomatics*, *70*(1), 38–43. 10.1159/000056223

Michalska, A., Szejko, N., Jakubczyk, A., & Wojnar, M. (2016). Niespecyficzne zaburzenia odżywiania się – subiektywny przegląd [Nonspecific eating disorders – a subjective review]. *Psychiatria Polska*, *50*(3), 497–507. 10.12740/PP/59217

Mikołajczyk, E., & Samochowiec, J. (2004a). Cechy psychologiczne pacjentek z zaburzeniami odżywiania w porównaniu ze studentkami wyższych szkół medycznych badanych kwestionariuszem EDI [Personality characteristics of female patients with eating disorders compared to female students of medical schools measured by the EDI questionnaire]. *Psychiatria Polska*, *38*, 170–171.

Mikołajczyk, E., & Samochowiec, J. (2004b). Cechy osobowości u pacjentek z zaburzeniami odżywiania [Personality characterisitcs of female patients with eating disorders]. *Psychiatria*, *1*(2), 113–119.

Morgan, J. (2000). From Charles Atlas to Adonis Complex—Fat is more than a feminist issue. *The Lancet*, *356*(9239), 1372–1373. 10.1016/S0140-6736(05)74051-4

Olivardia, R. (2001). Mirror, mirror on the wall, whos the largest of them all? The features and phenomenology of muscle dysmorphia. *Harvard Review of Psychiatry*, *9*(5), 254–259. 10.1080/713854919

Owsiejczyk, A. (2007). Determinanty kulturowe zaburzeń odżywiania [Cultural determinants of eating disorders]. *Roczniki Socjologii Rodziny*, *18*, 201–216.

Połom, M. (2015). Syndrom gotowości anorektycznej a struktura motywacji osiągnięć u uczennic szkoły średniej [Anorexia readiness syndrome and structure of achievement motivation among secondary school girls]. *Polskie Forum Psychologiczne, 20*(2), 184–200. 10.1456/PFP20150203

Pope, H., Gruber, A., Choi, P., Olivardia, R., & Phillips, K. (1997). Muscle dysmorphia: An underrecognized from of body dysmorphic disorder. *Psychosomatics, 38*(6), 548–557. 10.1016/S0033-3182(97)71400-2

Pope, H., Gruber, A., Mangweth, B., Bureau, B., deCol, C., Jouvent, R., & Hudson, J. (2000). Body image perception among men in three countries. *American Journal of Psychiatry, 157*(8), 1297–1301. 10.1176/appi.ajp.157.8.1297

Pope, H., Katz, D., & Hudson, J. (1993). Anorexia nervosa and "reverse anorexia" among 108 male bodybuilders. *Comprehensive Psychiatry, 34*(6), 406–409. 10.1016/0010-440X(93)90066-D

Pope, H., Phillips, K., & Olivardia, R. (2002). *The Adonis complex*. Simon & Schuster.

Schier, K. (1993). Rola symbolu w terapii psychoanalitycznej pacjentów w okresie dorastania [The role of symbols in psychoanalytical therapy of adolescent patients]. *Nowiny Psychologiczne, 3*, 103–108.

Stochel, M., Janas-Kozik, M., Zejda, J., Hyrnik, J., Jelonek, I., & Siwiec, A. (2015). Walidacja kwestionariusza ORTO-15 w grupie młodzieży miejskiej w wieku 15–21 lat [Validation of ORTO-15 Questionnaire in the group of urban youth aged 15–21]. *Psychiatria Polska, 49*(1), 119–134. 10.12740/PP/25962

Thompson, J. K., & Altabe, M. N. (1991). Psychometric qualities of the figure rating scale. *International Journal of Eating Disorders, 10*(5), 615–619. 10.1002/1098-108X(199109)10:5%3C615::AID-EAT2260100514%3E3.0.CO;2-K

World Health Organization. (1993). *The ICD-10 classification of mental and behavioural disorders*. World Health Organization.

Zięba, A., Bury, E., Kędzierska, E., Orzelska-Górka, J., & Gibuła-Bruzda, E. (2018) Preparaty hormonalne w dopingu wydolnościowym [Hormonal substances in performance doping]. In J. Bednarski, M. Bajda, M. Pawlicka, K. Bałabuszek, A. Mroczek, A. Kobyłka, K. Kasprzak, A. Szopa, K. Wojtunik-Kulesza, & A. Nogalska (Eds.), *Nauki Przyrodnicze i Medyczne: Żywienie, Sport oraz Zdrowie* [Environmental and health sciences: Eating, sport, and health] (pp. 98–117). Instytut Promocji Kultury i Nauki.

Ziółkowska, B. (2000). Uwarunkowania ekspresji syndromu gotowości anorektycznej [Determinants of Anorexia Readiness Syndrome (ARS) expression]. *Studia Minora Facultatis Philisophicae Uniwersitatir Brunensis, P4*, 35–55.

Ziółkowska, B. (2001). *Ekspresja syndromu gotowości anorektycznej u dziewcząt w okresie adolescencji* [The expression of the anorexic readiness syndrome in adolescent girls]. Wydawnictwo Fundacji Humanjora.

Ziółkowska, B., & Wycisk, J. (2010). *Młodzież przeciwko sobie. Zaburzenia odżywiania i samoouszkadzenia – jak pomóc nastolatkom w szkole* [Youth against themselves. Eating disorders and self-harming behaviors – how to help adolescents in school]. Wydawnictwo Difin.

5 Clinical diagnosis of personality structure and body image in patients with anorexia, bulimia, and binge eating disorder

The psychological (psychodynamic) diagnosis of personality structure maturity allows for refining the clinical assessment of the specific body image distortions (which are related to the personality structure). Among the significant indices for personality structure diagnosis (defined within the psychodynamic approach) are the specific psychological traits and body image (body Self) distortions characteristic for eating disorder patients simultaneously displaying varied personality structures: neurotic, borderline, or psychotic. Medical and pharmacological care are joined with a multifaceted psychotherapy adapted to the developmental capabilities of the patient's personality structure and the related levels of distortions in experiencing one's own physicality.

Personality structure and body image: the psychodynamic perspective in diagnosis and psychotherapy

The psychological diagnosis of the personality structure and its maturity may constitute a significant complement to the nosological diagnosis of eating disorders and may also clarify the clinical assessment of specific body image distortions. Thus, treatment of patients with anorexia or bulimia can be more effective from the very beginning, as medical care and pharmacotherapy will be combined with comprehensive psychotherapy adapted to the developmental possibilities of the patient's personality structure and the related level of body image distortions.

The self-harming behaviors in eating disorders concern both the attitude toward food and nutrition as well as the attitude toward physical activity. In each case, the attitudes center around the self-destructive nature of behaviors aimed at the body, as they are influenced by emotional and cognitive body image distortions and the desire to have a socioculturally promoted, low body mass index (BMI). Generalizing the whole spectrum of various body image definitions, disorders in this area can be considered to include the imagery, thoughts, and emotions which together evoke dissatisfaction with and lack of acceptance of one's own body (Cash, 2004; Cash & Smolak, 2011). A negative attitude toward the body and the discrepancy between the

DOI: 10.4324/9781003251088-5

actual and ideal body image are based on low self-esteem, which leads to various self-harming behaviors, including restrictive eating, intensive physical activity, or compulsive purging. Aside from body dissatisfaction, the psychological features of patients with anorexia or bulimia that are particularly often indicated in the literature include perfectionism (especially in anorexia), impulsivity (especially in bulimia), low interoceptive awareness (difficulties in adequate reception of physiological stimuli), inadequate self-esteem, and difficulties in building emotional bonds and relationships with others (Garner, 2004). In eating disorders, the body often symbolically expresses repressed internal conflicts, difficulties, and emotional disorders. Regardless of a medical diagnosis of a given eating disorder, each patient also has a specific personality structure. Distorted perception and negative thinking about one's own body (negative body esteem) as well as body dissatisfaction may be experienced and presented by patients with anorexia or bulimia in slightly different ways depending on the destabilization of psychological mechanisms of the neurotic, borderline, and psychotic personality structure (Cierpiałkowska & Górska, 2016; Cierpiałkowska & Soroko, 2017; Clarkin et al., 2013; Gabbard, 2015).

Contemporary medical classifications of eating disorders and personality disorders (ICD-10 and DSM-V) mainly focus on the descriptive symptoms and do not allow for a comprehensive psychological diagnosis (Cierpiałkowska & Marszał, 2013). From the perspective of evidence-based practice in medicine and clinical psychology (American Psychological Association, 2006 after: Cierpiałkowska & Sęk, 2016), psychoanalytical theories and object relations theory indicate the etiology and psychological mechanisms influencing the development of pathological personality structures (Cierpiałkowska & Górska, 2016). Object relations theory, in particular Otto Kernberg's structural and developmental model of the organization of the personality structure, provide the basis for the diagnosis of different levels pathology in personality organization (Cierpiałkowska & Górska, 2016; Cierpiałkowska & Soroko, 2017; Gabbard, 2015).

Kernberg's theory-based model of personality organization was developed in 2006 by the American Psychological Association (American Psychological Association, 2006, after: Cierpiałkowska & Sęk, 2016). Diagnosing the psychodynamic organization of the personality structure based on object relations theory allows for the analysis of the relationship between the mental disorder symptoms and the specific personality structure on the one hand, and the medical diagnosis of neurotic, psychotic, and/or personality disorders on the other (Cierpiałkowska & Marszał, 2013; Kernberg, 1996; Kernberg & Caligor, 2005). Kernberg's model of personality structure describes the personality as a system that undergoes continuous transformation of the self-representation in relation to the object, from the symbiotic period to separation and individuation, and toward the development of mature defense mechanisms (from primitive ones, e.g., splitting and projective identification, to neurotic ones, e.g., repression, suppression, and sublimation; Kernberg, 1996). Personality may be characterized by different levels of integration: from poor integration dominated by primitive defense mechanisms (the borderline organization) to a well-organized neurotic structure (with neurotic defense mechanisms predominating; Caligor & Clarkin, 2013; Gabbard, 2015; Kernberg & Caligor, 2005).

The psychodynamic diagnosis of the personality structure organization is a significant complement to the medical diagnosis of eating disorders based on the ICD-10 and DSM-V criteria because the proposed psychodynamic clinical criteria do not contradict the diagnostic indicators of personality dimensions proposed by the authors of the Big Five concept – Costa and McCrae (Grabski & Gierowski, 2012). Moreover, they supplement the DSM-V criteria. Kernberg's structural–functional model of personality characterizes the differences between the borderline, psychotic, and neurotic personality structure referring to the following diagnostic dimensions: (a) the specificity of the defense mechanisms, (b) the level of identity integration, and (c) the ego's ability to test reality (Clarkin et al., 2013; Gabbard, 2015). A person with anorexia or bulimia may present a neurotic, borderline, or psychotic personality structure. The different functional dynamics of psychological mechanisms (both defensive and adaptive) in each of these three personality structures may influence the direction of psychotherapy and, consequently, effectiveness of treatment in this group of patients. Therefore, apart from recognizing the treatment indications resulting from the nosological diagnosis of anorexia or bulimia according to the ICD-10 or the DSM-V criteria, it is also worth considering the specificity of the personality structure of a given patient. It can be assumed that the greater the destabilization of the personality structure in patients with eating disorders, the greater the escalation of self-destructive attitudes and behaviors toward the body and self, and the greater the difficulties in building emotional bonds with others.

Patients with anorexia and bulimia present specific psychological profiles of self-destructive attitudes and behaviors toward their own body corresponding to the intensity of disturbances in the development of their personality structure. The destruction of the body occurs through malnutrition. Apart from the already-formed mental Self, the patients' personality structure also includes the body Self (Krueger, 2002a, 2002b). The body Self is the basis for the development of the mental Self and it shapes the emotional and cognitive experience of one's own body in anorexia or bulimia. Patients with anorexia or bulimia have numerous emotional defects in the cognitive experience of the body (negation of the body), as well as defects in the perception of interoceptive stimuli, including hunger and satiety. Taking into account the importance of the psychological diagnosis of personality in determining the course of psychotherapy of eating disorders, the psychodynamic diagnosis of the personality structure, regardless of the nosological diagnosis, should also be considered.

In the process of diagnosis and treatment, it is worth taking into account the psychological indicators of personality structure destabilization, namely,

1   the patient's manner of reality testing (i.e., adequacy in perceiving the world, oneself, one's own identity as well as the boundaries of one's own body);
2   the patient's control of emotions and impulses;
3   the patient's pattern of establishing relationships with others (including distrust and uncertainty in interpersonal relationships and in building emotional bonds with others).

Based on the psychodynamic diagnosis, it can be assumed that the level of organization of the personality structure of patients with eating disorders is also expressed through the specific psychological features and attitudes toward the body. The level of harm (exhaustion) caused to the body through the intensification of the mental and somatic disease symptoms may vary based on the patient's personality structure. The stability (maturity) of the personality structure – neurotic or nonneurotic (borderline or psychotic) – may also affect how patients will experience and exhibit those psychological features and attitudes toward the body in specific behaviors.

Therefore, when making a clinical diagnosis of the psychological features of patients with eating disorders, it is worth considering both the specific psychological features as well as the personality structure (Fig. 5.1).

In order to complete the description of the psychological profiles of patients with eating disorders from the perspective of clinical diagnosis, it is worth pointing to the significance of the personality structure.

The neurotic personality structure and body image: diagnostic indicators

Based on the subject literature, the psychological figure of the neurotic personality structure is most often characterized by:

•   A stable structure of the ego and the superego (no identity pathology and no blurring of boundaries; a stable, not excessively punishing superego).
•   Internal conflict and disorder on the level of the so-called Oedipal phase of development (within Freud's model of personality development).
•   Domination of neurotic defense mechanisms (so-called secondary, higher order, more mature mechanisms such as denial, regression, intellectualization, rationalization, moralization, sexualization, acting out, reaction formation, identification, sublimation, etc.) relating to the person's internal boundaries (e.g., between the id, ego, and

Body image diagnosis	Diagnosis of the early childhood bonds pattern of emotional neglect and psychological trauma	Psychodynamic diagnosis of personality structure

• The level of pressure and internalization of sociocultural standards of the body image

          → The neurotic level

• The identity and strength of the ego (testing reality and recognizing the boundaries between the external and internal world)

          → The borderline level

• The strength and type of dominant defence mechanisms

• Level and type of self-destructive behaviors

          → The psychotic level

• A pattern of building bonds and relationships with other people

DIAGNOSIS OF PSYCHOLOGICAL TRAITS

Dissatisfaction with the body appearance

Assessment of the sense of physical fitness of the body and care for physical fitness

Perfectionism   Low self-esteem   Fear of gaining weight

Interpersonal distrust and difficulties in social relations   Interoceptive Deficits   Bulimic thinking, impulsiveness   Fear of maturity (adulthood)

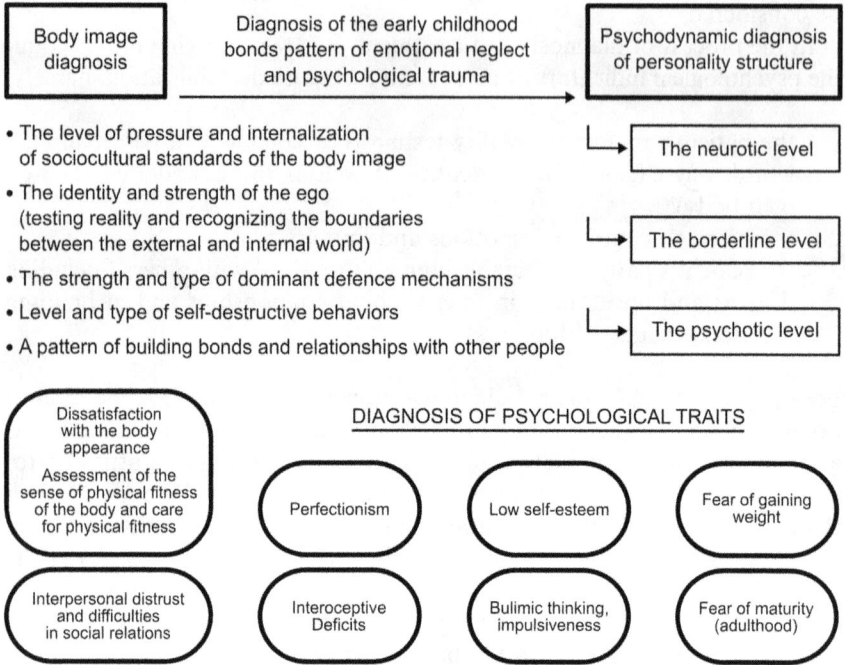

Figure 5.1 Model of clinical diagnosis of specific psychological features of patients with eating disorders. Source: own elaboration.

superego, or between the observer's ego and the experiencer's ego). In particularly stressful situations, neurotic people may use primitive defense mechanisms, but they are rather an exception to the dominant use of denial (Gabbard, 2015).

Patients with eating disorders who present the neurotic level of the personality structure have an integrated sense of identity, which causes relatively consistent behavior and an ego-dystonic experience of eating disorder symptoms and attitudes toward the body. In this case, the symptoms and the resulting behavioral difficulties also become unwanted. There are no disturbances in the patients' relationship with reality, as the conflict takes place internally (rather than externally, between the patient and others). The internal conflict is dominated by themes of separation and individuation (i.e., emotional separation from the family and entering into adulthood and independent life). Compared to patients with severe personality disorders, patients with eating disorders have less intense cognitive and emotional body image distortions and do not exhibit extreme perfectionist tendencies. However, they do exhibit increased impulse control (higher interoceptive awareness and simultaneously less intense experience of emotional states).

The self-observing ego present in the neurotic personality structure gives the eating disorder patients the opportunity to recognize the disorder and its related difficulties, meaning that the patients have the ability to obtain cognitive and emotional insight into the psychological mechanisms of the disorder. People with the neurotic personality structure are also characterized by the presence of an internalized (intrapsychic) conflict concerning contradictory, unconscious desires, impulses, needs, and feelings. The conflict is mostly between the id and the superego. In response, unconscious neurotic defense mechanisms are usually activated. In this case, eating disorder symptoms (restrictive weight loss and intensive physical activity, body dissatisfaction, obsessive thinking about food, eating, and body weight, bulimic cycles, i.e., binging and purging) are used to reduce anxiety and internal tension. Psychoanalytical concepts indicate clearly occurring relationships between the neurotic symptom and the unconscious internal conflict. The symptom is not accidental, but rather is "embedded" in the symbolism of the neurotic personality structure. A neurotically "embedded" eating disorder symptom is different from restrictive dieting, physical exhaustion, binging and purging, and various somatic ailments. Patients with anorexia, bulimia, or binge eating disorder simultaneously presenting the neurotic personality structure symbolically express fears related to:

- the superego (feeling guilt when standards cannot be met);
- castration (loss of genitals, other, body parts, or other injuries);
- losing the love or approval of a significant object;
- separation (loss of the object as such).

On the other hand, such patients show a lower intensity of persecutory fears (of invasion of hostile objects and annihilation) and fear of disintegration (loss of self, boundaries, internal cohesion; Clarkin et al., 2013; Gabbard, 2015). These, in turn, seem to be more prominent in patients exhibiting deeper personality psychopathology (borderline or psychotic). When patients with anorexia, bulimia, or binge eating disorder present deeper personality disorders, the configuration of psychological traits and attitudes related to the body, and thus the intensity of anti-health behaviors, change (Izydorczyk, 2015).

Patients with anorexia or bulimia who present the neurotic personality structure usually have an integrated sense of identity. Their behavior is relatively consistent and adequate to the stimuli being acted upon, except for the desire for an idealized body image. In this case, there is a significant discrepancy between the subjective assessment of body image and the real body image, described by the BMI. Patients with anorexia or bulimia and the neurotic personality structure experience a strong fat phobia and desire an idealized body image (i.e., lower BMI). As it dominates in neurotic people, the so-called ego-dystonic experience of eating disorder symptoms and attitudes toward the body means that the symptoms and the resulting difficulties are experienced as strange and unwanted (Gabbard, 2015). The patients do not present identity disorders (they test reality correctly; they show no disturbances in orientation in time or space). In addition, they have the ability to experience the state of internal conflict, and they are able to become aware, within the therapeutic process, of the unconscious content of the conflict.

The internal conflict most often experienced by such patients involves unconscious difficulties in the process of separation and individuation. Compared to patients with profound personality disorders (borderline and psychotic), patients with the neurotic personality structure have less severe cognitive and emotional body image distortions. They do not show extreme obsessive–compulsive and perfectionistic tendencies in relation to the body (e.g., fasting, extreme diets, or intensive physical exercise). On the other hand, they show preserved impulse control and, therefore, lower impulsivity toward the body (e.g., purging, self-harm, addictions). Instead, anxiety or depressive reactions appear more often, possibly with further impulse limiting and control. Patients with the neurotic personality structure also have higher interoceptive awareness (more accurate recognition and responses to experienced emotional states), which allows working on destructive impulse control behaviors. The self-observing ego present in the neurotic personality structure gives such patients the opportunity to recognize the specificity of their disorder and the resulting emotional difficulties. They have the ability to reflect on their own mental states and to gain cognitive and emotional insight into the psychological mechanisms of the disorder (Cierpiałkowska & Górska, 2016; Cierpiałkowska & Soroko, 2017; Gabbard, 2015).

Patients with the neurotic personality structure are characterized by the presence of an internalized (intrapsychic) conflict regarding contradictory unconscious desires, impulses, needs, and feelings. In response, unconscious neurotic defense mechanisms (e.g., denial, suppression, rationalization, intellectualization, reaction formation, and others) are usually activated. The eating disorder symptom (restrictive weight loss and intensive physical activity, body dissatisfaction, obsessive thinking about food, eating, and body weight, bulimic cycles, i.e., binging and purging) reduces anxiety and internal tension. In this way, the neurotic patients regain control over the own body and the sense of its limits.

Psychoanalytical concepts indicate clear relationships between the neurotic symptom and the unconscious internal conflict. Among eating disorder patients with the neurotic personality structure, the conflict most often revolves around such content as disgrace, incompetence, imperfection, criticism, rejection, and unattractiveness. In turn, they feel the need for uncritical support, acceptance, love, and safety, they fear humiliation, ridicule, rejection, evaluation, criticism, anxiety, and tension, and they do not take risks or attempt new activities. They remain in an unconscious conflict between the need for love and distrust, between the desire to self-actualize and doubts about own competences. Having a well-formed ego ideal, high aspirations, and a strong need for self-realization, but also a strong, punishing superego, they enter into social relationships and build emotional bonds with others only after making sure that they are safe and completely accepted (Cierpiałkowska & Soroko, 2017; Gabbard, 2015).

Summarizing the above, it can be concluded that among patients with eating disorders, the neurotic personality structure – compared to deeper personality pathology – includes correct reality testing, a lack of identity disorders, and an adequate body schema (orientation in one's own body, experiencing its limits), a relatively low level of cognitive (thoughts and perceptions) body image distortions, low levels the sense of worthlessness, incompetence, distrust in interpersonal relations, low interoceptive deficits (higher level of impulse control), slightly increased perfectionism, and perceived fear. Body idealization, fat phobia, and body dissatisfaction are present, but without extreme (without psychological insight) negation of own body.

Borderline and psychotic personality structures and body image: diagnostic indicators

In reference to the psychodynamic paradigm and the classification provided by Otto Kernberg (Cierpiałkowska & Marszał, 2013; Clarkin et al., 2013; Gabbard, 2015) and Nancy McWilliams (2014), profound personality disorders are most often encountered in people with the so-called borderline and psychotic personality structures. Due to a great similarity with the mentioned people and between the borderline and the psychotic personality structure in terms of primitive defense mechanisms, the characteristics of the functioning of both those structures are presented together below. However, it is worth pointing out the psychotic personality structure is characterized by a greater intensity of primitive defense mechanisms (especially projective identification and splitting, including fragmentation of the self) than the borderline structure, as well as a greater risk of quicker psychotic decompensation (Gabbard, 2015). Both personality structures also occur among patients with eating disorders, for example, in highly restrictive anorexia with the dominance of symbiotic and obsessive–compulsive features. In bulimia, the borderline personality structure is more common.

The primitive defense mechanisms used by patients with the borderline and psychotic personality structures include withdrawal, denial, omnipotent control, primitive idealization, projective identification, dissociation, and splitting. Defense mechanisms relate to the boundary between the Self and the outside world, are formed in the preverbal development stage, and are automatic. Therefore, they are not subject to the reality principle, but rather operate in a global, undifferentiated manner (Clarkin et al., 2013; Gabbard, 2015; McWilliams, 2014). The conflict is external, taking place between the Self (ego) and the outside world. A primitive personality organization, poorly organized ego, fear of annihilation, persecution fears, and intense idealization dominate. From a developmental perspective, in interpersonal relationships, patients with eating disorder initiate transference. Then, splitting and projective identification dominate instead of denial. The thinking of such patients is "influenced by an emotional defect" (Gabbard, 2015). They are dominated by aggressive and self-aggressive behaviors, and high impulsivity causes fear (suicidal and self-harming behaviors, substance use, etc.), chaos, disjointed or fragmented speech, and instability in relationships – difficulties in managing relationships on the verbal and emotional level. Moreover, such patients reveal clearly defined affect, weak ego boundaries, fears of the destructive potential of their own feelings, fears of insufficient or excessive closeness, and a varied but usually significant defect in the personality structure (the ego).

Eating disorder symptoms are experienced ego-syntonically (as something typical, natural, and inherent). An important element differentiating between the neurotic and the borderline and psychotic personality structures is also the level of control over impulses, body image, and interpersonal relationships. In both personality and eating disorders, body image distortions and body image control constitute strong reinforcers. They lead to excessive perfectionism and, thus, debilitating drive for thinness. On the other hand, due to the destabilization of the borderline personality structure, a characteristic feature of bulimia is the loss of control over own behavior, impulses, and drives. The pleasure of self-development and realization of desires and drives is replaced by the satisfaction with perfect control and denial of "common pleasures." Interpersonal conflicts are transferred to the body and food. Fat phobia increases and provokes many unconscious fears, anxieties, and unresolved internal conflicts concerning self-esteem, self-efficacy, and a sense of security in the world.

Specific defense mechanisms and body image

A characteristic defense mechanism in this group of patients and at this level of personality structure destabilization is splitting (Gabbard, 2015; McWilliams, 2014). It concerns a variety of objects: family members, hospital staff, food, body parts, thinking, feelings, and so forth. Splitting in relation to food is common to all eating disorders – on the one hand, food is a valuable object that is stored (stolen, given to others, sometimes patients even sleep with food in their beds). Food gains a special value, like substances in addiction. On the other hand, unlike in addiction, food is also an evil object that should be purged from the body as soon as possible through vomiting or enemas. Food is a good object, while eating itself is bad. Splitting also involves the body. On the one hand, the body is a valuable object that must be perfect (hence the frequently observed intensive physical exercise). On the other hand, the body is unacceptable in its natural (mature, sexually developed) form. An important element is also the splitting between the body and the mind (Izydorczyk, 2015; Józefik, 1999; McWilliams, 2014).

In the mind-body dimension, the mind is more valuable, and the body only interferes with it. For the anorexic patient, the body is a "thing" and the mind is a "person" (subject). In the patient's fantasies (not always conscious), as the "thing" grows, the "person" disappears. Splitting leads to the internal division into parts, which is reflected in the patients' relationships with the social environment and with the body. For example, in the patients' fantasies, individual organs are presented as good or bad, and this is how the patients experience them. They are independent of the person of the patient. They feel insecure and describe their condition as "fragmented." Patients with eating disorders try to control their body (by fasting, purging, and intensive physical exercise), which contains objects that are experienced as dangerous. The patients also develop a hidden system of fantasies about the body, in which it becomes significantly distorted. The patients see their body as monstrous, obese, swollen with food, heavy, impossible to move around, and so forth.

In addition to splitting, projective identification (projecting internal, evil, vengeful, or persecutory objects and trying to control them in external objects) is also a significant defense mechanism in patients with borderline and psychotic personality structures (Clarkin et al., 2013; Gabbard, 2015; McWilliams, 2014). Here, the body and food become the evil, persecuting objects. Projective identification is connected with the blurring of the Self's boundaries, revealed when patients "feed others" to feel sated themselves. Another defense mechanism is denial. Patients with eating disorders and deeply destabilized personality structures deny their needs and experiences in many areas of life: the need to eat and to maintain their own appearance, experiences of somatic stimuli, the eating disorder itself, and their difficulties in relations with objects (e.g., the mother). They also deny some of their own behaviors, such as purging or stealing food (which is then stored and often used to vomit).

In sum, the immaturity of the psychological mechanisms in the borderline and psychotic personality structures in patients with anorexia and bulimia means that they will present equally immature and primitive patterns of emotional, cognitive, and social responses to their own body (based on splitting and projective identification). Chaos and impulsivity are among the dominant features of the cognitive and emotional attitude to the body. Patients with anorexia and bulimia show a pronounced affect, weak ego boundaries, fears of the destructiveness of their own feelings, fears of insufficient or excessive closeness, and a varied, but usually significant defect in the personality structure, which causes disturbances in reality testing as well as inadequate emotional reactions. Moreover, such patients usually also experience disturbances in adequately perceiving their own body boundaries and strong cognitive (thoughts and perceptions) body image distortions (the body is often perceived as a "monster"). They engage in various forms of self-mutilation, suffer from various addictions (drugs, alcohol, medications, etc.), have very low self-esteem (in bulimia, and in anorexia, repressed under feelings of omnipotence and idealization), a strong sense of incompetence, as well as distrust and difficulties in interpersonal relationships.

References

American Psychological Association (2006). APA Presidential Task Force on evidence-based practice (2006). Evidence-based practice in psychology. *American Psychologist*, *61*(4), 271–285. 10.1037/0003-066X.61.4.271

Caligor, E., & Clarkin, J. (2013). Model osobowości i patologii osobowości oparty na teorii relacji z obiektem [The object relations model of personality and personality pathology]. In J. F. Clarkin, P. Fonagy, & G. O. Gabbard (Eds.), *Psychoterapia psychodynamiczna zaburzeń osobowości* [*Psychodynamic psychotherapy of personality disorders*] (pp. 23–61). Wydawnictwo Uniwersytetu Jagiellońskiego.

Cash, T. F. (2004). Body image: Past, present, and future. *Body Image*, *1*(1), 1–5. 10.1016/S1740-1445(03)00011-1

Cash, T. F., & Smolak, L. (2011). Understanding body images: Historical and contemporary perspectives. In T. F. Cash, & L. Smolak (Eds.), *Body image: A handbook of science, practice, and prevention* (pp. 3–11). The Guilford Press.

Cierpiałkowska, L., & Górska, D. (2016). *Mentalizacja z perspektywy rozwojowej i klinicznej* [*Mentalization from a developmental and clinical perspective*]. Wydawnictwo Naukowe UAM.

Cierpiałkowska, L., & Marszał, M. (2013). Patologia organizacji osobowości w teorii relacji z obiektem O. Kernberga [Pathology of personality organization in O. Kernberg's object relations theory]. *Czasopismo Psychologiczne*, *19*(1), 47–56.

Cierpiałkowska, L. & Sęk, H. (2016). *Psychologia kliniczna* [Clinical psychology]. PWN.

Cierpiałkowska, L., & Soroko E. (Eds.). (2017). *Zaburzenia osobowości. Problemy diagnozy klinicznej* [*Personality disorders. Issues in clinical diagnosis*]. Wydawnictwo Naukowe UAM.

Clarkin, J. F., Fonagy, P., & Gabbard, G. (2013). *Psychoterapia psychodynamiczna zaburzeń osobowości* [*Psychodynamic psychotherapy of personality disorders*]. Wydawnictwo Uniwersytetu Jagiellońskiego.

Gabbard, G. (2015). *Psychiatria psychodynamiczna w praktyce klinicznej* [*Psychodynamic psychiatry in clinical practice*]. Wydawnictwo Naukowe Uniwersytetu Jagiellońskiego.

Garner, D. M. (2004). *EDI-3. Eating Disorders Inventory. Professional Manual.* Psychological Assessment Resources, Inc.

Grabski, B., & Gierowski, K. (2012). Zaburzenia osobowości-różne spojrzenia i próby ich integracji [Personaltiy disorders – various approaches and integration attempts]. *Psychiatria Polska*, *46*(5), 829–844.

Izydorczyk, B. (2015). *Postawy i zachowania wobec własnego ciała w zaburzeniach odżywiania* [Attitudes and behaviors towards the body in eating disorders]. PWN.

Józefik, B. (Ed.) (1999). *Anoreksja i bulimia psychiczna. Rozumienie i leczenie zaburzeń odżywiania się* [Anorexia and bulimia. Understanding and treatment of eating disorders]. Wydawnictwo Uniwersytetu Jagiellońskiego.

Kernberg, O. F. (1996). A psychoanalytic theory of personality disorders. In J. F. Clarkin, & M. F. Lenzenweger (Eds.), *Major theories of personality disorders* (pp. 106–140). The Guilford Press.

Kernberg, O. F., & Caligor, E. (2005). A psychoanalytic theory of personality disorder. In M. F. Lenzenweger, & J. F. Clarkin (Eds.), *Major theories of personality disorders* (pp. 114–155). Guilford Press.

Krueger, D. W. (2002a). Psychodynamic perspective on body image. In T. F. Cash, & T. Pruzinsky (Eds.), *Body image. A handbook of theory, research, and clinical practice* (pp. 30–37). The Guilford Press.

Krueger, D. W. (2002b). *Integrating body self and psychological self. Creating a new story in psychoanalysis and psychotherapy*. Bruner-Routledge.

McWilliams, N. (2014). *Diagnoza psychoanalityczna [Psychoanalytic diagnosis]*. Gdańskie Wydawnictwo Psychologiczne.

6 Psychotherapy of body image distortions in patients with eating disorders: an integrative approach

The integrative approach in psychotherapy shows the need to use scientifically documented – in line with evidence-based practice – combinations of elements of psychotherapy specific to different schools, which results in an individualized approach to therapy of patients with various mental disorders, including eating disorders. Psychotherapy in the integrative approach introduces the possibility of flexible and evidence-based treatments. In the case of body image distortions in patients with eating disorders, it is worth pointing to the usefulness of integrating psychodynamic psychotherapy techniques.

Nonspecific and specific therapeutic factors in psychotherapy of body image distortions from the perspective of psychological theories

Models of psychotherapy are dominated by a holistic and transdiagnostic approach. They emphasize the importance of multifaceted therapeutic influences on the mechanisms of disorders rather than only focusing on symptom reduction and narrow nosological diagnosis. Psychological diagnosis of body image distortions, including the psychodynamic diagnosis of the personality structure, is an element of a holistic approach to eating disorders and is simultaneously consistent with evidence-based practice (American Psychological Association, 2006, qtd. in: Cierpiałkowska & Sęk, 2016). It allows for adjusting the direction of psychotherapy to fit the pattern of the patients' behavior toward their body displayed in accordance with their personality structure. In all eating disorders, the common basic pathology concerns the nature of the cognitive structures, especially the perceptual and cognitive body image distortions. In the light of the psychiatric/psychological literature, the etiology of eating disorders is often considered in the psychoanalytic–psychodynamic paradigm, in particular the British (Klein, Winnicott) and American object relations theories (Mahler, Kernberg, Kohut). Their authors point to the importance of object relations both in the development of disturbances in separation and individuation as well as in ego development of patients with eating disorders (Glickauf-Hughes & Wells, 1997; Grzesiuk, 2005).

DOI: 10.4324/9781003251088-6

According to these concepts, the quality of the early childhood matrix of the relationship between the child and the mother (or other primary caregiver) has a significant impact on the later pattern of forming adult relationships. This is especially true of the therapeutic relationship. There, the therapist often assumes the role of an emotional container, a mother-object through which a group or individual therapeutic process can develop. The basic assumptions of Klein's theory as well as Bruch's developmental approach to eating disorders emphasize the importance of the specificity of the development of early childhood, nonverbal communication between the child and the mother (Bruch, 1971, 1983) in their pathogenesis. Incorrectly understanding the child's nonverbal signals, the mother is unable to identify and adequately satisfy the child's needs. Thus, in their place, the child introduces his own needs as dominant. The mother's ideas about the child are not verified, and the boundaries between her fantasies about the child's unmet needs and reality become blurred.

From a psychodynamic and developmental perspective, eating disorders represent a maladaptive solution to a number of dilemmas and internal conflicts accompanying the period of maturing and entering adulthood. Most often, these conflicts cannot be resolved because they are cut short by "turning off" the drives – biologically "killing" them, for example, by starvation. Instead of playing out in interpersonal relationships, they are "shifted to food and body."

Object relations theorists emphasize the importance of early emotional bonds that are significant in shaping character and later emotional and social relationships. The concept of corrective interpersonal experience and insight into the psychological mechanisms underlying the relationships with others are important points of reference in therapy of eating disorders (Glickauf-Hughes & Wells, 1997).

Representatives of the British and American object relations schools suggest that treatment should focus on understanding the patient's inner world of representations by diagnosing repeated patterns of interactions with others and providing the patients with a therapeutic (corrective) relationship that would enable them to solve the ego split (Glickauf-Hughes & Wells, 1997). Sullivan (2001), a representative of the American interpersonal school, also indicated the importance of the therapeutic relationship in helping the patients create a coherent Self system and improve their interpersonal relationships. As can be seen, emphasizing the interpersonal relationships and relationships with significant objects in both individual development and treatment is a chief point in many therapeutic approaches (Grzesiuk, 2005).

According to Fairburn (2013), therapy is supposed to restore the patient's ability to fully and directly enter into contact with people. In therapy, the patients become aware of the "bad" internalized objects that were once necessary for their functioning. The therapist becomes a "good enough" real object so that the patient can break ties with the bad objects.

Therefore, the therapist should not arouse guilt and shame in the patient (Glickauf-Hughes & Wells, 1997; Grzesiuk, 2005). Object relations theorists (e.g., Mahler, Winnicott) pointed out that for therapy to help the patients develop their true self, it should:

- recreate a sufficiently good maternal environment, so as to fill the deficits that led to the development of a false Self;
- induce a controlled regression, in which the patient returns to the period of unfulfilled early needs and errors of the environment and reacts to them appropriately;
- provide sufficiently good maternal and environmental functions that the patient did not experience in childhood (Glickauf-Hughes & Wells, 1997; Grzesiuk, 2005).

Kohut's self-psychology also emphasizes the importance of internalized relationships for personality and Self development. According to Kohut, the child's Self develops through the interaction between his innate potential and the parents' reactivity, pointing to the importance of a good (empathetic) mother for the development of the true Self. The creation of a therapeutic relationship based on empathy allows for activating the patients' primary developmental problems, gives them the opportunity to idealize the therapist or use them as a mirror, a kindred soul, and allows for the expression of large-scale fantasies, which makes them more conscious and available for therapy (Glickauf-Hughes & Wells, 1997; Grzesiuk, 2005).

Kernberg formulated specific treatment indications depending on the level of the patient's character pathology. He drew attention to the combining of partial images of the Self and the object within therapy (especially with patients with more severe disorders), so that patients can create "multidimensional, coherent and integrated images of [themselves] and others" (Kernberg, 1996). In addition, he pointed out the importance of confronting the patients with their negative transference and primitive defense mechanisms, especially unprocessed, strong aggression. Kernberg postulated the structuring of the therapeutic session to minimize acting out behaviors (see Glickauf-Hughes & Wells, 1997). The psychodynamic approach to mental disorders and psychotherapy indicates strengthening ego functioning and the corrective emotional experience as important therapeutic goals (Grzesiuk, 2005). To achieve them, it is vital to establish a positive therapeutic relationship from the very beginning of treatment. The patients' unconscious defense mechanisms (including projective identification, splitting, denial, and idealization) and phenomena of transference and countertransference play an important part in this process. Their negative and unconscious nature often makes it impossible to quickly establish a stable therapeutic relationship. Anorexic patients with the psychotic personality structure (with strong symbiotic and anankastic patterns of cognitive and emotional attitudes toward the body, eating, and relationships) usually reveal an excessive attachment to controlling their body shape and weight, and, therefore, to controlling eating (to reduce body weight and maintain a desired physical appearance). From the perspective of psycho-dynamic diagnosis, the basic psychological mechanisms underlying the borderline and psychotic personality structures determine the emerging eating habits that are subordinated to rigid and restrictive rules (diets, physical activity, and compensatory behaviors, i.e., various forms of pur-ging). On the one hand, the pattern of establishing a positive emotional relationship becomes important as a condition for building a therapeutic alliance during the initial phase of treatment. On the other hand, therapeutic work on the cognitive and emotional reconstruction of the pattern of the relationship with the body is required. In that case, therapeutic techniques typical of the cognitive–behavioral and psychodrama approaches (presented below) are useful. In line with the above theses of the psychodynamic ap-proach to diagnosis and psychotherapy, the main assumptions of cognitive and cognitive–behavioral theories indicate improperly shaped (in the course of learning) cognitive structures (cognitive concepts) or habits (behavioral concepts) as significant determinants of eating disorders and body image distortions. Significant distortions in the perception of and thought patterns about the body in anorexia or bulimia require cognitive restructuring (i.e., teaching new, adaptive ways of thinking) for recovery (i.e., reduction of and symptoms and disorder processes).

The proven effectiveness of cognitive–behavioral therapy in the treatment of eating disorders is also combined with the use of psychoeducation and dietary support (especially in the initial phase of treatment; Jaworski et al., 2017; Lewitt et al., 2008). This particularly concerns expanding the patient's knowledge in the field of rational nutrition, psychological and physiological consequences of hunger, and the metabolic needs of the organism. Here, the perspective of nutritional education correlates with the regulation of body image distortions because it favors learning corrective (pro-health, i.e., not harmful) behaviors toward the body.

At the initial stage of treatment, the specificity of the patients' personality structure, life history, and previous emotional experiences in relations with relatives (parents, siblings, etc.) and the social environment (peers) is not immediately known. The level of personality structure destabilization (neurotic and deeper, including psychotic), as well as the experienced and established patterns of emotional responses in relationships (based on early childhood experiences in family relationships) affect the quality of the de-veloping transference (positive or negative) and the therapeutic relationship (Gabbard, 2015; Grzesiuk, 2005). If the patient begins therapy while in a state of physical exhaustion (i.e., heart rhythm disturbances, critical body weight), treatment will usually take place in strictly monitored, inpatient circumstances. In such a situation, psychotherapeutic work on increasing awareness of internal conflicts underlying the eating disorder becomes meaningless. Such patients are so physically exhausted that they are unable to mentally work and use their emotional resources. Psychological help in regulating behaviors toward the body in the event of cachexia often requires supporting the patient's decision to agree to hospitalization, which is not always readily accepted and which may arouse resistance and opposition. Due to many pathological psychological mechanisms (denial, primitive idealization, omnipotent control, splitting, projective identification, rationalization, intellectualization), patients with anorexia, not only of the restrictive type, block/cut off their emotional experience of the body and they cognitively distort (through schemas and perception) their perception of their body image (Iniewicz et al., 2002; Józefik, 1999; Józefik et al., 2002).

Patients with anorexia see themselves differently than their doctors, psychologists, psychotherapists, and relatives (parents, siblings, partners, colleagues, friends, etc.) who have an accurate assessment of their psychophysical state. The patients' lack of identification with the disorder and the resulting cognitive distortions do not allow for a realistic assessment of the destructive effects of one's own functioning. Therefore, when the patients' self-aggressive approach to the cognitive and emotional experience of the body comes to the fore in the treatment (body dissatisfaction, restrictive drive for thinness, increased perfectionism), it becomes important for the developing transference to have a positive character and for the countertransference to include impulses often marked by hostility and negation of the relationship (Clarkin et al., 2013; Gabbard, 2015; Izydorczyk, 2017; McWilliams, 2014). Most often, they are related to the patients' experience of their body and treating (as a result of projection) others as wanting to harm the patients by denying them the perfect body image. The patients defend their (most often distorted) body image and attitude. At a conscious level, they do not understand the specificity of their own internal conflict, which is unconscious and related to the world of emotional experiences (Gabbard, 2015; Iniewicz et al., 2002; Izydorczyk, 2017; Józefik, 1999; Józefik et al., 2002). Usually, the externally or passively (hidden) explored aggression and aversion in relation to the therapist is associated with a transference reaction, internal factors (personality traits, e.g., perfectionism), and defense mechanisms (e.g., denial, splitting, projective identification, blocking of emotions, rationalization). Therefore, at the initial stage of treatment, a positive therapeutic relationship is fundamental for further building an alliance in therapy, also with regard to working on the patient's experience of physicality (Clarkin et al., 2013; Grzesiuk, 2005; Izydorczyk, 2017).

Experiencing positive emotions in the therapeutic relationship favors this process and simultaneously supports the acquisition of a negative attitude toward the harmful anorexic or bulimic symptoms by the patient. These symptoms are to a large extent dynamized by a distorted (cognitive) body image, its emotional nonacceptance, drive for thinness, and fat phobia. Therefore, the therapeutic relationship established on the basis of positive transference provides the vehicle to arouse positive emotions and adaptive thought patterns in the patients in relation to their own body (Grzesiuk, 2005; Izydorczyk, 2015, 2017).

The use of unconscious processes (positive transference and counter-transference analysis) from the outset of treatment, may support the process of acquiring new (constructive, i.e., not based on cognitive distortions and emotional negation) knowledge about the body and stimulate new behaviors, for example, by changing the perception of and attitudes toward regular weight control by the medical personnel. Usually, it causes fear and avoidance in the patients, and agreeing to regular weight control is one of the basic parts of the therapeutic contract in the treatment of eating disorders. If the patients unconsciously develop an emotionally positive matrix of relations with the doctor or therapist, it might be easier for them to accept a confrontation and (despite resistance) agree to regularly weigh themselves as well as monitor other symptoms (induced vomiting and other forms of purging, binge eating, etc.). Often, patients argue with the medical staff and demand explanations why they need to be weighed, questioning the correctness of the specialists' decisions. In addition, they ask for the right to refuse the weight measurement. Usually, with an empathetic but firm, rational, and confrontational explanation of the doctor or therapist's position, as well as with the developing positive transference, it is possible to maintain regular weighing. In this context, the body and its protection are considered from the perspective of the patients' relationship with their body and their (emotional and cognitive) attitude toward it, as well as from the broader perspective of the patient's body and others' attitudes toward it (the doctor or therapist's interventions show how important it is for them personally, as well as from the perspective of treatment). As a result of the confrontation with reality and real requirements, a "new matrix" of a gradually developed relationship with the body may be formed.

Phenomenological and humanistic psychotherapy also offer similar perspectives to psychodynamic work with the patients and their body (Grzesiuk, 2005). These approaches see the source of the disorder in the accessible content of human consciousness: distorting the image of oneself and the surrounding reality. Disorders are treated in terms of deficits in personality development resulting from the failure to meet the essential psychological needs (i.e., love, acceptance, autonomy, and realization of important values). The goal of therapy is thus to create conditions for the corrective emotional experience for the patient, as the body is inseparable from the spiritual side of existence. In Gestalt therapy, the "here and now" is the basis for working with the patients' experiences in contact with their body. The energy of the organism, blocked by the disorder, is evident by the inhibition of emotional expression in relations with others (Grzesiuk, 2005). This is often reflected in bodily symptoms (e.g., voice modulation, facial expressions). The lack of contact with one's own feelings manifests itself as a lack of consistency between the spoken words and body language. The methods of working with the body in psychodrama and Gestalt therapy are similar to psychodynamic ones, although they have a different function (they are aimed at experiencing the body "here and now" and deepening the sensations flowing from it). Among the most important therapeutic factors is the quality of the therapeutic relationship, a significant part of which is founded on authenticity, empathy, and unconditional acceptance of the patient by the therapist (Grzesiuk, 2005). It also stimulates positive emotions and increases the motivation for therapy in the initial phase, later supporting the acquisition of new experiences and practice of new behaviors (e.g., related to food). In the case of patients with eating disorders, this plays an extremely important role, because such a therapist attitude often shows the patients a model of behavior based on nondirectiveness, empathy, and authenticity which stands in contrast to their perfectionist and/or compulsive behavior patterns (Grzesiuk, 2005). Such therapeutic attitude does not preclude authentic and empathetic confrontations regarding the therapeutic contract, for example, in the case of regular body weight control or other medical examinations (e.g., measuring the frequency of purging).

Alexander Lowen (2020) presents an interesting, original approach to psychosomatic disorders which highlights the importance of the body in their etiology and treatment. Moreover, his approach is consistent with the assumptions of psychodynamic and humanistic approaches. The source of the disorders is the chronic emotional tensions resulting from unresolved intrapsychic conflicts. In this concept, life is an energetic process based on breathing. The bodily symptoms such as muscle stiffness signal the body's energy level. The condition for the harmonious development of the body and mind is the so-called anchoring in the body (i.e., free contact – experiencing every part of the body) and grounding (i.e., the free flow of energy through the body toward the ground). Bioenergetic exercises are used in order to restore balance and free the patient from the experienced emotional tension. These include massages, stretching, diaphragmatic breathing, and teaching the patient to adopt the correct body posture that will restore the flow of sensations. In order for eating disorder patients to engage in such exercises, they must cooperate with a therapist. Establishing a constructive therapeutic relationship from the very beginning of treatment is thus necessary. It will allow for the therapist to work on the patients' contact with their body, increasing their abilities to learn new (healthy) behaviors toward the body.

Summarizing the basic theoretical assumptions from the perspective of treating body image distortions, it is worth indicating the following universal therapeutic guidelines.

1. Depending on the identified indicators of body image distortions in anorexia, bulimia, or binge eating disorder, it is worth considering the multifaceted and multidirectional interactions in the therapy plan: from the psychodynamic approach to cognitive–behavioral techniques, psychoeducation, psychodrama, and family therapy and counseling.

2. Both nonspecific and specific therapeutic factors play a role in each stage of treatment. Multidirectional interactions which depend on the adopted theoretical paradigm are taken into account in the comprehensive (medical, psychotherapeutic, dietary) treatment process of eating disorders. Each adopted paradigm (e.g., psychodynamic, cognitive–behavioral, humanistic–existential, systems) determines the interventions used in treatment aimed at recovery. This also means correcting the cognitive and emotional disturbances in the patients' own experience of their physicality.

3. Treatment of eating disorders carried out in accordance with the standards of modern scientific (medical and psychological) knowledge should use the specific (medical and psychotherapeutic activities planned in accordance with the theoretical paradigm describing the mechanisms of the disorder and the process of therapy) as well as the nonspecific (universal) factors supporting therapy (Czabała, 2006). These include:

    *   fostering a sense of security and positive emotions in the therapeutic relationship, as well as supporting adequately negative emotions and attitudes in relation to previous and current life experiences;
    *   focusing the therapeutic relationship on building cooperation (an alliance between the patient and the therapist/doctor);
    *   acquiring new knowledge and practicing new skills and behaviors.

4. Nonspecific therapeutic factors, universal between the theoretical paradigms, indicate the need to build a positive emotional relationship between the patient and the therapist/doctor as the basis for establishing a therapeutic alliance. Thus, this is a starting point for further therapeutic actions and changes: changes in the patients' attitude toward their body as well as real, concrete changes in their life. The therapeutic relationship provides the basis for acquiring new knowledge that, by training new (corrective) behaviors toward the body, leads to change. The therapeutic relationship between the patient and therapist is of significant importance all throughout the treatment.

5. In addition to nonspecific therapeutic factors based on a positive therapeutic alliance and relationship, it seems necessary to take into account the appropriate specific therapeutic factors depending on the patient's personality structure and psychological profile.

6. In the first stage of therapy, when building the therapeutic alliance and motivation for treatment (i.e., toward achieving a healthy body mass index [BMI] and body image), attention should be paid to the psychological diagnosis of the patients' body image (their experience of own corporeality) and the psychological determinants of their behaviors toward it, as well as to supporting the development of pro-health motivation for treatment.

7. The first stage of treatment is a turning point in the patients' everyday life. It is usually challenging because the patients begin to identify with the disease to a greater or lesser extent (even if they do not directly declare it and are not aware of it). Usually, with a more or less unstable motivation to undertake treatment, the various (usually still not entirely conscious) specific psychological mechanisms underlying the eating disorder also need to be addressed. Regardless of the personality structure and body image distortions, the patients require a similar treatment (focused on similar goals).

8. At the beginning of treatment, nonspecific (universal) healing factors referring to the empathic relationship between the patient and the therapist/doctor, based on authenticity and openness, are of central importance. They are recognized as significant in all therapeutic approaches. The elements of psychoeducation, cognitive–behavioral therapy (focused mainly on building motivation to establish a therapeutic contract regarding regular body weight control and medical examination), and psychological diagnosis also gain significance.

9. The positive attitude of the patient toward the therapist often requires empathy and openness (honesty) from the therapist because an excessively directive (authoritarian, associated with the dominant parent) attitude provokes the patient's resistance and withdrawal from the relationship. Patients with eating disorders are distrustful and sensitive to insincere social situations and relationships. They try to control the situation and carefully listen to the messages conveyed to them. They require honesty in mutual communication.

10. When building the therapeutic alliance, the initial stage should include the diagnosis of the specific emotional, cognitive, and behavioral body image distortions. The timing of introducing diagnostic measures depends on the nature of the therapeutic relationship as well as the therapist's skill.

Body image distortions in the neurotic personality structure: directions of psychodynamic therapy

In accordance with the standards of modern scientific (medical and psychological) knowledge, the recovery-oriented treatment of patients with eating disorders should use both nonspecific and specific therapeutic factors. Body image distortions are related to diverse personality structures. Clinical evaluation of the intensity of self-harming behaviors and the underlying psychological mechanisms of the neurotic, borderline, and psychotic personality structures should be considered when selecting therapeutic strategies (Clarkin et al., 2013; Gabbard, 2015; Kernberg, 1996; McWilliams, 2014). Each of these personality structures represents a specific, differentiated configuration of psychological and sociocultural factors shaping the body image, which determine the strength of self-harming (restrictive, impulsive) behaviors toward the body (Izydorczyk, 2015).

The specific constellation of sociocultural and psychological determinants (internal conflict in the process of separation and individuation), the specificity of the emotional and cognitive body image, and the resulting self-harming behaviors in patients with the neurotic personality structure warrant different directions of treatment in the area of body image than in the case of patients with the borderline or psychotic personality structures. According to object relations theory (Cierpiałkowska & Marszał, 2013; Gabbard, 2015), it can be assumed that eating disorder patients with borderline and psychotic personality structures will present a much higher level of psychopathology in the body Self (body image) and will experience their own body in a more self-destructive way. Patients with the neurotic personality structure are more often suitable for psychodynamic and insight-oriented psychotherapy (individual or group), while patients with the borderline or psychotic personality structures will benefit more from long-term psychodynamic psychotherapy due to the necessity of building the therapeutic relationship over a longer period of time (Clarkin et al., 2013; McWilliams, 2014).

The features distinguishing eating disorder patients with the neurotic personality structure with regard to their experience of the body are: lack of excessive impulsivity, preserved stable ego boundaries, preserved ability to test reality, and the ability to adequately experience both pleasant and unpleasant somatic stimuli. Due to the specificity of the neurotic personality structure in patients with eating disorders (neurotic and mature defense mechanisms combined with the developed ability to cope with stress), they are more suited for insight-oriented therapy which includes deepening the insight into the psychological mechanisms (internal conflicts) behind body image distortions (Clarkin et al., 2013; Gabbard, 2015). Eating disorder symptoms (restrictive weight loss, fasting, intensive physical exercise, binging, and purging) are a symbolic reflection of internal conflicts transferred onto the body. Body image distortions (negation of own body despite a healthy BMI) in patients with the neurotic personality structure is often significantly influenced by internalized sociocultural body image standards. They are related to the sexualization of the female body (Fredrickson & Roberts, 1997) and the phenomenon of westernization, namely, the cultural universalization of body image standards promoted in western cultures (Izydorczyk et al., 2019; Izydorczyk et al., 2020). Individual or group insight-oriented psychodynamic therapy is a process in which patients with eating disorders, due to the neurotic personality structure and specific configurations of psychological features, along with the current strong body dissatisfaction, are able to cope with and follow therapeutic interventions.

Psychodynamic insight-oriented therapy in the treatment of body image distortions

The body Self is the basis for the formation of the mental Self (Krueger, 2002a, 2002b). The specificity of the psychological determinants of anorexia, bulimia, and binge eating disorder usually warrants complex and multi-stage interventions aimed at searching for the unconscious causes of the symptoms, body dissatisfaction, and the associated fat phobia. When patients with eating disorders have established a therapeutic relationship with the therapist, focus can shift toward understanding the origin of the symptoms and interpersonal difficulties. Why are the patients dissatisfied with their life? Why do the patients dislike their body and refuse to accept the fact that they are destroying it and risking their life? There are many more questions, but they chiefly revolve around the need to recognize the underlying unconscious conflicts and emotional deficits (most often experienced in interpersonal relationships). Different typologies of personality disorders, defense mechanisms, perfectionism, and fat phobia may increase the patient's resistance toward becoming aware of unresolved internal conflicts and suppressed emotions as the main sources of body image distortions. Psychodynamic insight-oriented psychotherapy, both in individual and group format (apart from the obvious differences resulting from group dynamics), assumes that the symptoms of various mental disorders have similar psychological sources (Grzesiuk, 2005). Symptoms of eating disorders usually perform specific, symbolic functions expressing psychological mechanisms similar to many other disorders. The more the pattern of behaviors toward the body is based on extrinsic (sociocultural) stimulation and the neurotic personality structure, the easier (faster) it is to build a therapeutic alliance and begin psychodynamic work on insight into the psychological mechanisms of body image distortions, namely, understanding the causes behind the symptoms of overeating, restrictive weight loss, or the use of other compensatory behaviors.

In addition to fostering insight into the psychological sources of the disorder (including cognitive and emotional body image distortions), psychodynamic interventions for eating disorders are often aimed at compensating for the patient's basic emotional deficits and resolving the internal conflicts (Izydorczyk, 2015; Józefik, 1999, 2014). Based on the patient's past experiences and current clinical material, the therapist works with the patient to understand the underlying psychological mechanisms of eating disorders and body image distortions.

In the context of the neurotic personality structure, the psychodynamic interventions (clarifications, confrontations, and, above all, interpretations) address both the body Self (schema, perceptions, thoughts, and emotions related to the body, interoceptive awareness of the body in relationship with oneself and others, and the socioculturally shaped attitude toward the body) and the mental Self (psychological mechanisms of the personality structure). Taking into account the above-mentioned complexity of body image factors in eating disorders and recognizing the specificity of the emotional difficulties in building a therapeutic alliance (usually a strongly developed, fear-driven need for excessive control), it is worth considering the use of cognitive–behavioral elements in the initial phase of treatment (see sections below on "cognitive–behavioral therapy in the treatment of body image distortions" and Chapter 7; Carnabucci & Ciotola, 2013; Fairburn, 2013).

In the initial stage of treatment, the patients adapt to the situation through the therapist's exploring questions and psychoeducational interventions which may focus them on further work on their feelings, attitudes, behaviors, and social relations related to the body image. The relatively short duration and the verbal character of the dialog in a psychodynamic group or individual session does not make it easy for patients to quickly "warm up" to work on their internal conflicts and explore the psychological sources of the eating disorder symptoms. In addition, when working with compulsively overeating and overweight patients, depending on their individual needs, it is also worth considering cognitive–behavioral therapy with elements of psychoeducation (Fairburn, 2013). For overweight women, nutritional and dietary interventions will be important to achieve a controlled reduction of above-average body weight and prevent obesity. Such patients do not display increased compensatory behaviors (purging) and instead use overeating as an emotional regulation strategy. The patients must understand why they overeat, as it is the key to changing their body image. Due to the importance of emotional and social support and the introduction of corrective social modeling, it is worth considering group therapy for such patients. They often have negative experiences in peer contacts, a low sociometric position, low self-esteem, and low body esteem. On the other hand, the dynamics of the group process (therapeutic alliance and relationship with the group, support, sense of community) are important therapeutic factors modifying the patient's existing experiences and sociocultural patterns of behavior toward the body (Grzesiuk, 2005; Summers & Barber, 2014).

In addition to the positive role of group mechanisms, insight-oriented therapy also allows for identifying areas of unconscious conflicts based on the fear of maturation/adulthood as the main sources of self-harming restrictive and bulimic behaviors. Due to the patient's specificity of current functioning, the preserved ability to reflect on internal experiences, and the level of psychopathology, group psychodynamic psychotherapy can be an important inspiration for change (Summers & Barber, 2014). Enriching it with elements of body work can additionally support this process. It is also worth to remember the importance of building a therapeutic relationship with the patient and assuming an educational attitude that would introduce the patient to the treatment from the position of authority (without pressure, but with clearly clarified rules and conditions for recovery).

In addition to the basic assumptions of the adopted theoretical paradigm, BMI control, medical examinations, and assessments of the patient's psychophysical state should be incorporated into treatment from its initial phase (to a varying degree, depending on the type of eating disorder and personality structure). In patients with the neurotic personality structure, including weight control in the therapeutic contract is less important, because they do not usually suffer from body wasting. However, the more dominant the medical and psychological indicators of eating disorders, the smaller the opportunities for using psychotherapeutic interventions. Thus, hospitalization becomes obvious as a basic condition of treatment. In such situations, due to other therapeutic goals, the therapist supports the patient's motivation to agree to a medical consultation and hospitalization. Therapeutic activities during this time are related to the need to understand the patients' emotional situation on the one hand and to confront the patients with the real risks to their health and life on the other (especially if the patients engage in intensive self-harming behaviors). The therapist's task is to help the patients realize the extent of the risk to their health and the possible risk of death. Confrontation is thus both necessary and difficult. This is particularly important in the case of patients with high levels of destructive perfectionism and impulsivity who engage in frequent and varied self-harming behaviors (Izydorczyk, 2015; Józefik, 1999). Taking an educational attitude toward the patient whose symptoms are worsening serves the primary goal of this stage of treatment. A clear message from the therapist that the patients are unable to make a realistic assessment of their body weight, level of exhaustion, and general health (which poses a threat to their life) is simultaneously an offer to support them in the process of regaining health and determining the terms of the therapeutic contract.

Body image distortions in the borderline and psychotic personality structures: directions of psychodynamic therapy

Significant deficits in interoceptive awareness, strong impulsivity and/or perfectionism, and distrust and uncertainty in interpersonal relationships (significant difficulties in building emotional bonds with others) occurring in patients with eating disorders and the borderline and psychotic personality structures significantly hinder the process of insight-oriented therapy from the outset (Clarkin et al., 2013; Gabbard, 2015). Due to the psychosomatic nature of eating disorder symptoms, the patients in long-term group therapy are obliged by the therapeutic contract to undergo medical examinations, maintain or increase their body weight, and undergo medical examinations (Jaworski et al., 2017). During treatment, the patients are held accountable for following the contract. Taking responsibility for the patients and alleviating their compulsion of excessive control is a reversal of their original relationship with the mother (the patient is not supposed to take care of the group and the therapist's wellbeing at his own expense; rather, the group and the therapist care for the patient). Setting requirements to the patient (closely related to the body) and enforcing the contract is also often met with resistance. This resistance requires analysis and reformulation, that is, entering into a relationship based not on struggle, but on empathetic understanding. In this process, it is also important to set firm boundaries, which the patients did not experience often in the childhood relationship with their parents. Clear boundaries on the part of the therapist are of particular importance for patients who are emaciated and who engage in binging and/ or purging behaviors (Izydorczyk, 2017).

Treatment with overly perfectionist and controlling patients (most often diagnosed with restricting anorexia, binge eating and purging anorexia, or bulimia) should constantly center around the question of: when do self-harming behaviors and attitudes dominate and how to encourage the patients to fight for their life? A therapeutic relationship should be built, but when the patients are not aware of their distorted (cognitively and emotionally) image of their body and the health consequences of their self-harming behaviors, the therapist with whom they are voluntarily working, at least on the declarative level, becomes a mirror reflecting the patient's real (self-destructive) state (Izydorczyk, 2017). In the first phase of treatment, special attention should be paid on establishing the therapeutic contract determining the medical and physical criteria (e.g., BMI) necessary to safely proceed with psychological treatment. The patient's consent to regular weight control and medical examinations is an important point that allows the therapist to safely disengage from controlling the patient's somatic state and safely focus on symptom reduction. The symptoms are based on entrenched psychological features, for example, perfectionism, high deficits in interoceptive awareness, low body esteem, a tendency toward obsessive thinking about food, and distrust in interpersonal relationships. Weight control is particularly important in anorexic patients suffering from cachexia. The configuration of their psychological features is not conducive to the treatment process, as it increases resistance and passive aggression toward oneself and others. Only when the patient has gained the psychological possibility of building relationships, using social support, and gaining a sense of security and trust, and is ready to reduce the excessive control over food and the body, treatment can focus on facilitating insight into the psychological mechanisms of the eating disorder.

Due to the different emotional and cognitive body image distortions and the difficulties in building a therapeutic alliance in eating disorders (presented in sections below – "nonspecific and specific therapeutic factors in psychotherapy of body image distortions from the perspective of psychological theories" and "body image distortions in the neurotic personality structure – directions of psychodynamic therapy"), long-term psychodynamic therapy based on building an emotional bond, with work on insight beginning later, is indicated for patients with the borderline and psychotic personality structures (especially the latter; Clarkin et al., 2013; Gabbard, 2015). Secondly, due to the previously described specific features of the borderline and psychotic personality structures as well as body image distortions, it is worth considering the incorporating cognitive–behavioral and psychodrama elements into the treatment process (Carnabucci & Ciotola, 2013; Fairburn, 2013). As was already mentioned, the borderline personality structure is associated with significant emotional and cognitive body image distortions which may require long-term cognitive restructuring (i.e., changing in order to more adequately correspond to reality). Apart from long-term psychodynamic psychotherapy, cognitive–behavioral and psychodrama techniques can also be helpful in this process (Carnabucci & Ciotola, 2013; Fairburn, 2013).

The specificity of psychodynamic therapy and psychodrama as an integrative approach have been presented in the section below – "cognitive–behavioral therapy in the treatment of body image distortions." Thus, this chapter presents the specificity and importance of long-term therapy of eating disorders based on the therapeutic relationship. The specificity and intensity of transference and countertransference among patients with eating disorders and the borderline or psychotic personality structures indicate the need for long-term psychodynamic therapy centered around building a therapeutic relationship (also including work on body image distortions). Such patients often describe the sensations flowing from their body as a confusing conflict (Carnabucci & Ciotola, 2013). In symbolic language, this type of relationship with the body can be described as "a battlefield between different sensations" that the patient experiences also in the relationship with the therapist. The subjective experience of the patients who often cuts off their own emotions and experiences through the defense mechanisms of splitting or projective identification, is usually connected with the therapist feeling similar bodily sensations and emotions. The patient's feelings are often characterized by a lack of integration of various interoceptive stimuli. This happens, among others, due to the predominance of splitting and the transference and countertransference based on the mechanism of projective identification (Clarkin et al., 2013; Gabbard, 2015; Izydorczyk, 2017). In feeling their own body, the patients often experience strong impulsivity or block emotions and interoceptive stimuli. Thus, treatment should start with building a corrective emotional bond before undertaking insight work aimed at emotional frustration through the interpretation of reflections on the sources of the symptoms. For such patients, insight work usually starts later than for neurotic patients. Moreover, the low level of interoceptive awareness confirms the necessity to simultaneously take into account therapeutic body work. From the psychodynamic and developmental perspectives, early developmental inhibition in shaping a stable, integrated, and coherent body image is the result of improperly assimilated emotional interactions with primary caregivers (Clarkin et al., 2013; Glickauf-Hughes & Wells, 1997; Krueger, 2002a, 2002b). The pathological consequences of this fact can be reduced to the elements of parental influence: (a) the dominant of interaction patterns (increased aggressiveness, hyperactivity), (b) the parents' empathetic inaccessibility, and (c) inconsistency and selectivity of reactions. The therapist's transference and countertransference are related to the patient's primary relationship pattern with the caregivers in childhood (Gabbard, 2015; Glickauf-Hughes & Wells, 1997; Krueger, 2002a, 2002b).

The psychodynamic understanding of the influence of parental behavior on disruptions in body experience emphasizes the negative impact of parental control and overprotection as well as the expectations for the child to adapt to the parents' standards. This causes developmental inhibitions in the area of body experience. The body is perceived as blurry, weak, childish, asexual, undifferentiated, and mixed with the image of the parents. The parents' empathetic availability is lacking, that is, when the parents are unable to react accordingly to the child's emotions, physical sensations, and behaviors, the child's experience does not become a point of self-reference. The parents' inconsistent reactions to select stimuli from the child create a selective reality (e.g., the mother may ignore emotional and kinesthetic stimuli, responding only to physical needs or physical pain).

The mother's response pattern teaches the child to perceive and organize his experience in such a way as to gain attention and provoke reactions. Efficiency is associated with the body. experiencing the body and mental Self through pain and discomfort becomes deeply rooted in the child's personality and interaction patterns, creating a predisposition for the psychosomatic style of expression (Krueger, 2002a, 2002b). If the development of a complete and clear body image is inhibited, later attempts to develop it may be associated with sensory overstimulation to ensure that the body is felt and experienced (e.g., excessive exercise in anorexia, self-harm, binge eating, substance abuse, risky behaviors).

Long-term psychodynamic therapy based on the therapeutic relationship in the treatment of body image distortions

Having experienced disorders in the development of the body Self in early childhood, many patients with eating disorders and the psychotic or borderline personality structures feel their body as something separated from them, which can be easily interfered with. They may try to overcontrol it, creating a specific image of the body and themselves through intensive physical exercise, fasting, or abrupt weight gain. In patients with a dominant impulsive pattern of emotional regulation (associated mainly with bulimia and the binging and purging type of anorexia), bulimic behaviors (binging and purging) may result from the need to create the boundaries for the external body image and basic body experience (Izydorczyk, 2015). Actively trying to define the boundaries of the body may also include such behaviors as irritating the skin, wearing loose clothes to feel a scratchy sensation, compulsive masturbation and sexual behaviors, weight gain, and self-harm. Stimulation of interoceptive awareness can be achieved by binging and purging behaviors or the sensations associated with excessive physical exercise. In the above-described patterns of emotional regulation associated with behaviors toward the body, the use of cognitive–behavioral therapy techniques (psychoeducation, cognitive insight into sociocultural messages) as well as family therapy and counseling (e.g., pointing to the impact of transgenerational messages and family myths on body image) may not be enough to lead to emotional and cognitive insight or changing the harmful behavior patterns (Józefik, 2014).

Apart from cognitive–behavioral therapy elements (in response to empathetic inaccessibility on the part of the parents), the corrective emotional bond with the object (therapist) becomes important in working on reducing self-destructive behaviors (Fairburn, 2013). For this reason, in many situations, long-term individual psychodynamic therapy is needed to provide the basis for such an experience (Clarkin et al., 2013; Summers & Barber, 2014). Increased perfectionism and its dominant role in provoking self-harming behaviors toward the body warrants individual contact and time to build a therapeutic relationship rather than short-term therapeutic interactions in the cognitive–behavioral paradigm. Patients with anorexia and the psychotic personality structure (with its symbiotic and obsessive–compulsive features) as well as strong behavioral overcontrol may not be able to constructively engage in group psychotherapy (especially in the medium- and short-term psychodynamic approach).

One alternative may be long-term group psychotherapy, in which activities are largely focused on building relationships. "Proud," overcontrolling patients with anorexia, strongly separated from their emotions and perfectionist, will have difficulties with "giving up control" by "showing emotions." It is easier for the therapist to gain access to the displaced and blocked emotional experiences through a direct, empathetic relationship. Therefore, in the entire course of treatment of body image distortions in patients with the psychotic personality structure, the dominant role of building the therapeutic relationship should be taken into account as the basis for acquiring corrective emotional experiences in relation to others and to one's own body (Summers & Barber, 2014). Insight in this area remains in the service of the therapeutic relationship. Together, introduced in the right order, it give the patients the opportunity to change their self-harming behaviors toward the body.

A slightly different way of functioning in the therapeutic relationship will be revealed by patients with bulimia and the borderline personality structure, usually presenting an impulsive pattern of relationships with their own body, food, and other people. Although such impulsivity also indicates significant psychological dysfunctions in the experience of the body, group therapy can be considered in addition to individual therapy. The impulsive behavior and expression of emotions allows for their exposure to the external environment. In group therapy, the group helps analyze the intragroup relations and assumed member, noting that the patients also recreate these roles in their current relationships outside the group. The group stimulates the search for the sources of destructive behaviors toward the body in past experiences. Through group dynamics and support, it is possible to work with the patients on their sense of internal cohesion and continuity – emphasizing that what used to be an adaptation is now an obstacle. The role of body image in the etiology of eating disorders plays a central role here. It is important to realize where the symptoms came from and what function they perform for the patient.

Psychodynamic group therapy creates a space where patients can experience and express various emotions, "discover" denied, unacceptable feelings and impulses, and learn about the richness and complexity of their inner world and how to respect it, which allows for a change in the maladaptive, pathological defense mechanisms toward a greater adaptation to the patients' real needs (Grzesiuk, 2005; Summers & Barber, 2014). The therapy group undergoes a corrective process of shaping and rebuilding identity through the search for internal rather than external points of reference for experiencing and understanding oneself as a separate individual. This also applies to experiencing the body as a subject, part of the Self. The role of the group in modeling new (corrective, pro-health, not driven by anxiety) behaviors toward their body is also important. Learning these new behaviors often causes resistance due to the rigidity in existing behaviors (binging and purging). In the psychodynamic understanding of the group process, the long-term group (the symbolic mother) can adjust itself in a corrective way to the level of social and emotional dysfunction of the members suffering from eating disorders (Clarkin et al., 2013). The role of the group is to contain the emotions of a given patient and to create an environment in which his psychological needs will be noticed, understood, and satisfied, unlike in the patient's previous relationships, which were an important element in the development of eating disorders (Krueger, 2002a, 2002b). The development of such an appropriately dependent, safe, and noninjurious relationship is the basis through which a good object will be internalized and will make possible the process of separation and individuation, which may further deepen insight into the psychological and sociocultural sources of the eating disorder.

As already mentioned, in addition to psychodynamic psychotherapy, treatment of patients with eating disorders and the neurotic, and especially borderline personality structures, cognitive–behavioral therapy techniques well-described in the literature (Fairburn, 2013) should be considered, along with operating techniques, psychodrama, and art therapy (Carnabucci & Ciotola, 2013).

Cognitive–behavioral therapy in the treatment of body image distortions

Correction of body image distortions, reducing restrictive and/or bulimic behaviors toward the body, and replacing them with healthy behaviors and habits are extremely important tasks in the treatment of eating disorders (Fairburn, 2013). In order to achieve change in the attitude toward the body, it is worth considering – according to the individual patient needs and the personality structure diagnosis determining the level of body image distortions – the use of operating techniques (i.e., cognitive–behavioral techniques and psychodrama). Below, the basic assumptions and goals of cognitive–behavioral and psychodrama techniques in working with the body image of patients with eating disorders will be presented.

Developing cognitive and emotional insight into the psychological mechanisms of eating disorders is usually not sufficient to fully remove the behavioral symptoms of body image distortions and attitudes toward food and eating. Patients with eating disorders often need additional therapeutic interventions in the cognitive–behavioral approach, implemented in a group or individual context. Usually, in the initial phase of treatment, psychoeducation and cognitive–behavioral techniques should be used. They support the pro-health motivation to start treatment and work on strengthening the therapeutic contract, simultaneously supporting work on reducing the discrepancy between the real and idealized body image which provokes strong dissatisfaction and body image distortions (Fairburn, 2013). This especially concerns treatment of patients with anorexia. The specificity and directions of using cognitive–behavioral techniques in the treatment of eating disorders are presented above (see above), where the differences in psychotherapy of body image distortions in patients with the neurotic and borderline personality structures were discussed, indicating the need to adjust psychoeducation and interventions to both. Cognitive–behavioral techniques are helpful in stimulating the patients to agree to medical examinations and regular weight control, and they indicate the significant role of social modeling in reducing anti-health behaviors toward the body and food (Carnabucci & Ciotola, 2013; Fairburn, 2013).

At later, more advanced stages of treatment (when the therapeutic alliance and relationship are established), cognitive–behavioral interventions are usually aimed at correcting cognitive and emotional body image distortions as well as the psychological mechanisms of the obsessive–compulsive bulimic cycle (binge eating and purging; Fairburn, 2013). Their use is particularly important in the treatment of patients with anorexia of the binge eating and purging type and bulimia, in whom the mechanisms of compulsive overeating intensify the cycles of bulimic symptoms.

An important category of interventions applied to these patients are the so-called nutritional interventions and psychoeducation toward proper nutrition (Jaworski et al., 2017). They are supported mainly by cooperation with a dietitian. These interventions have different meanings and goals in treatment of anorexia, bulimia, and binge eating disorder. Promoting healthy eating habits along with elements of cognitive–behavioral therapy (working with the body and the mechanisms of binge eating) will be important in patients with anorexia and bulimia and the neurotic, borderline, and psychotic personality structures. In patients with the neurotic personality structure who are strongly influenced by sociocultural body image standards, nutritional interventions and psychoeducation may become important in the first stage of treatment in order to support coping with the idealized body image and fat phobia. The patients are usually ashamed of their symptoms and experience them as ego-dystonic. At this stage of treatment, they try to reduce them, assuming that they will not gain weight. However, fat phobia makes it difficult for them to work on changing body image distortions if they are not supported in this area, for example, by a dietitian.

In patients with the borderline or psychotic personality structures, cognitive–behavioral interventions aimed at confrontation in the area of weight control and medical examinations may play a significant role throughout treatment (Fairburn, 2013). They are centered around enforcing physiological requirements of BMI, blood pressure, heart rate, or laboratory test results (e.g., electrolyte levels) control in order to continue psychotherapy. Usually, patients with restrictive weight loss diets have an obsessive "need to think about food," which generates significant anxiety. Giving in to one's own needs causes panic and dread so great that it takes the form of an eating phobia, an obsession with not eating/eating. Instead of eating, the patient realizes this need in fantasies of eating or feeding others. Weight loss is experienced as a success, it becomes proof of competence, strength, and endurance, while weight gain is failure, shame, and loss of self-control. Therefore, patients with anorexia have no choice but to deny that anything harmful is happening to them, because, paradoxically, the disorder may make give them a sense of self-worth. Up to a certain point, the disorder has more "benefits" than costs.

Introducing systematic monitoring of body weight and psychoeducation involves identifying self-harming behaviors and confronting them because the patient does not notice them or unconsciously displaces them. After building a therapeutic alliance and relationship and working on the patient's sense of security within it, it is also worth using psychoeducation and cognitive–behavioral interventions focused on learning and recognizing various environmental (situational) triggers of binge eating as well as reducing (or eliminating) binge eating and accompanying purging behaviors. An interesting intervention to reduce self-harming behaviors in patients with eating disorders may be the so-called bodywork group and symptom work group. This form of therapy is undertaken usually after completing psychodynamic therapy in order to consolidate and further develop the changes that have already been achieved. Working in a group that is homogeneous in terms of the members' diagnoses is based on a cognitive model of eating disorders that links the symptoms with the internal experiences, thoughts, most often of an automatic and self-destructive nature, and beliefs about oneself and others (expectations, obligations, intrapsychic, and interpersonal functioning). Education in distinguishing thoughts from feelings, as well as feelings and their physiological manifestations, introduces order into the patient's inner world and allows for greater coherence of the mental sphere, linking it with the somatic sphere. As a result, the symptoms are further psychologized and the disorder is externalized. The patient's identity can start developing apart from the symptoms.

Working on the symptoms of eating disorders in cognitive–behavioral group therapy, the patients further explore the sphere of needs and impulses and the cognitive development of difficulties in their expression, as well as search for strategies to satisfy these needs through other means than the "relationship with food" (Fairburn, 2013). In this way, it becomes much easier to resign from the symptoms, which are also understood as an intermediary object (preparation for this move lasts throughout the therapy, but it can take place on a conscious level from this point on). The patients also have the opportunity to reflect on the social determinants of their disorder, on their perception of their social role and the shaping influence of body image standards promoted in the media, and on the resulting expectations. This allows the patients to make more conscious choices and define themselves from a more independent position ("I want to be like that for myself, not for others"), which is related to a clearer identity and autonomy.

In anorexia and bulimia, the patients experience a series of splits: the bad body and the ideal mind, good and bad food. Their feelings also involve fragmentation of the body, expressed in the selective perception of certain features and omission of others, as well as in the inability to integrate and interpret stimuli from various sensory channels (visual, tactile, interoceptive). All sensory experiences that can activate drives and essential needs are cut off, starting with the most elementary ones – hunger, thirst, fatigue, cold, or sexual desire. The body is treated as an object that does not feel. The patient often expresses aggressive impulses which reflect an internalized, excessively strict and demanding parent, for example, by exercising for hours despite exhaustion. Therefore, the main goals of therapeutic bodywork are understood very broadly – from activating all sensory channels (sight, smell, temperature, hearing, touch), through focusing on interoceptive and proprioceptive stimuli, to paying attention to the feelings accompanying these experiences and trying to interpret their meaning. This allows the patients to learn to recognize their own needs as signaled by body sensations.

In addition, the tasks performed in the bodywork group concern learning relaxation and diaphragmatic breathing. The patients have the opportunity to take care of their body and control their emotions and drives (other than through fasting), while ignoring resistance. Dealing with the impulsive sphere should take place at a later stage of therapy, usually through visualizing and then reformulating that which was a source of shame or fear into something that gives opportunities for development. This allows for reducing negative attitudes toward sexuality or aggression.

An important aspect of therapy involves exercising and stimulating the recognition and defense of the body's (imagined and real) boundaries as well as the broader psychological boundaries, that is, the mental and physical need for distance and closeness.

In sum, the basic goals of bodywork using cognitive–behavioral techniques are: building a realistic body image, learning to experience pleasure in relation to the body, increasing awareness of the body's boundaries, and stimulating sensory awareness. Other, indirect goals of these interventions include developing social skills through learning to consciously use body language and practicing assertive behaviors (better impulse control, including tension relief). Due to the fact that patients with eating disorders participate in bodywork exercises and are in contact with a group of similar people, they learn to use body language, often neglected in their lives thus far. They can learn to notice the fact that the body can tell them a lot through nonverbal signals (e.g., pain, allergic skin reactions). The patients learn assertive behaviors (not aggressive, not dependent, but driven by acceptance and respect for themselves and others). This allows them to control activity and hyperactivity, improve their emotional self-control, and relieve frequently experienced tensions. The aim of bodywork is to teach the patients to experience pleasure in connection with the sensations flowing from the body.

Effective elements of psychoeducation include expanding the knowledge that restrictive fasting, diets, and suppression of naturally felt hunger also distort the proper perception of satiety. Additionally, stimulation of sensory awareness ("I have the insight that I experience my body, that I possess it") helps develop appropriate responses to stimuli coming from body parts and organs that often become "lost" in eating disorders. It should also focus on teaching the ability to adequately perceive such stimuli as hunger and satiety. Brain structures initially controlling this process are deprived of their "primary function" – instead of receiving signals from the body (hunger, leading to an appropriate cognitive interpretation and reaction), they stopped working according to the correct rules (Porges, 2020; Rosenberg, 2020). The patients cannot perceive real signals of hunger because they have been distorted by long-term attempts to ignore them by restrictive dieting or persistent (not consciously controlled) binge eating and purging. Cognitive–behavioral techniques in bodywork are most often used in a diversified way, adapted to the phases and forms (individual or group) of treatment as well as to the adopted theoretical paradigm and the patients' individual needs (in accordance with the specificity of their personality structure and body image distortions; Carnabucci & Ciotola, 2013; Fairburn, 2013). In the initial phase of treatment, apart from psychoeducation and interventions aimed at behaviors toward eating and the body, the following interventions are common:

- psycho-drawing of, for example, various types of human figure, often with a request to indicate the emotions experienced toward different parts of the body, to mark them with colors, to mark the parts associated with pain, suffering, ailments, and injuries in the past. This gives the patients the opportunity to reflect on their body image distortions (what body parts they omit from his drawing and which they inadequately exaggerate);

- visualizations: using imagination focused on themes related to body image, often in combination with music, rhythm, and symbols (exercises using projection and animal or nature symbols, e.g., selecting images of trees that best represent the current state of mind and attitude toward the body);
- active imagination: releasing associations in the form of creative physical movement;
- training in behaviors related to a healthy approach to experiencing the body and releasing emotional tension, for example, practicing safe contact with the body and experiencing stimulation (e.g., physical activity or passivity and relaxation);
- exercises stimulating and sensitizing interoceptive awareness (breathing and relaxation exercises) to build a realistic body image;
- movement and dance exercises: experimenting with body posture, providing space for experience of movement (defining and feeling the body's limits and boundaries, experiencing muscle tension and relaxation, awakening awareness of the body and its movement), experiencing the relationships between emotions and the body/posture;
- exercises deepening the awareness of hunger and satiety (relaxation and breathing exercises);
- exercises for passive motor mobilization (moving someone else's limbs);
- exercises in front of a mirror (confronting own appearance with the imagined one, creating an adequate body image).

Therapeutic work with the body in eating disorders: integration of cognitive–behavioral, psychodrama, and art therapy techniques based on the polyvagal theory

When searching for a scientific basis for therapeutic interventions related to the neutralization of emotional tension and introducing the feeling of "inner relief" necessary in treatment of eating disorders, and simultaneously related to body image and experience, it is worth pointing to Porges' polyvagal theory (2020). Interventions activating the vagus nerve and the neurobiology of the sense of security are examples of the possibility of integrating cognitive–behavioral, psychodrama, and art therapy techniques in treatment of eating disorders (Carnabucci & Ciotola, 2013). The relationship between the autonomic nervous system, especially the vagus nerve, and the internal organs shows the importance of the neurobiology of the sense of security in the treatment of post-traumatic stress disorder and other types of mental disorders with somatic symptoms. The polyvagal theory and the specificity of the vagal nerve indicates its significant connection with emotional states and behaviors (also toward the body). Porges (2020) also indicates the importance of the abdominal part of the vagus nerve as essential for rest, recuperation, physical and emotional health, and interpersonal bonding (Porges, 2020). Rosenberg (2020) points to the therapeutic significance of the vagus nerve in body-work. Referring to the polyvagal theory, in a situation of deprivation of the sense of security (e.g., psychological trauma and emotional deficits), the neurobiological basis of the abdominal part of the vagus nerve and the development of fight/flight reaction, depression, and emotional reactions are disturbed (Porges, 2020). Therapeutic assumptions based on the polyvagal theory introduced by Porges (2020) allow for using a spectrum of various nonverbal techniques in therapeutic bodywork: psychodrama (working with symbols), art therapy (especially music therapy and choreotherapy), and cognitive–behavioral therapy: psychoeducation and relaxation and meditation exercises. Carnabucci and Ciotola (2013) draw attention to the neurobiological foundations of the relationship with and the attitude toward one's own body, at the same time indicating the need to integrate verbal and nonverbal techniques (based on behaviors) in working body experience with patients with eating disorders. Carnabucci and Ciotola (2013) and Rosenberg (2020) also emphasize the influence of the brain and the peripheral nervous system on body experience, paying attention to the role of the vagus nerve (calling it the "smart vagus" nerve) in the mechanisms of eating disorders and their treatment. Restoring the ability to correctly perceive stimuli and emotions flowing from the body (e.g., stimulation of appropriate interoceptive awareness), working on "inner calm and emotional soothing," and restoring a sense of security (relaxation, meditation) are important tasks in working to reduce body image distortions in eating disorders. This is achieved by psychodrama techniques and interventions directly aimed at experiencing bodily stimuli and the physiological components of emotions (e.g., self-soothing – achieving an inner state of relief, relaxation, meditation, etc.; Carnabucci & Ciotola, 2013).

In verbal and nonverbal psychodrama techniques, it is important to build a sense of security in the treatment of eating disorders and work according to the rule that instead of forcing the body to act, one should listen to the body. Carnabucci and Ciotola (2013) emphasize that the determinant of changes in body image is behavior, not only verbal analysis. They also suggest that psychodrama and art therapy make it possible to use therapeutic techniques based on "experiencing and gaining inner consolation" in treating body image and experience distortions and self-harming behaviors symptomatic of eating disorders. The specific operation of the vagus nerve and the changes taking place in the brain due to of meditation, relaxation techniques, and psychodrama, choreotherapy (music therapy), and other techniques based on nonverbal "soothing" influence the brain areas related to empathy, memory, and the sense of self

(Rosenberg, 2020). They activate the presence of the "observing self" – the role of the witness – and therefore may be considered "soothing" behaviors. Through their nonverbal character, psychodrama techniques, and art therapy may enhance bodily relaxation and thus help/enable weaken the psychological mechanisms maintaining negative (self-harming) emotions toward the body in patients with eating disorders (Carnabucci & Ciotola, 2013).

In the integrative use of cognitive–behavioral techniques (especially relaxation exercises), psychodrama, and art therapy, symbols and playing metaphorical roles are especially important, for example, in working on diets and the patients' relationships with food and eating. A technique using metaphorical roles is the "self-soothing voice." Among similar techniques, there are also ones using rhythm and music, for example, the inner musician (melody improvisation; Carnabucci & Ciotola, 2013).

In a treatment of people with eating disorders it can be used verbal and nonverbal psychodrama techniques.

References

American Psychological Association (2006). APA Presidential Task Force on evidence-based practice (2006). Evidence-based practice in psychology. *American Psychologist, 61*(4), 271–285. 10.1037/0003-066X.61.4.271

Bruch, H. (1970). Psychotherapy in primary anorexia nervosa. *The Journal of Nervous and Mental Disease, 150*(1), 51–67.

Bruch, H. (1971). Death in anorexia nervosa. *Obstetrical & Gynecological Survey, 26*(11), 778–779.

Carnabucci, K., & Ciotola, L. (2013). *Healing eating disorders with psychodrama and other action methods. Beyond the silence and the fury*. Jessica Kingsley Publishers.

Cierpiałkowska, L., & Marszał, M. (2013). Patologia organizacji osobowości w teorii relacji z obiektem O. Kernberga [Pathology of personality organization in O. Kernberg's object relations theory]. *Czasopismo Psychologiczne, 19*(1), 47–56.

Cierpiałkowska, L. & Sęk, H. (2016). *Psychologia kliniczna* [Clinical psychology]. PWN.

Clarkin, J. F., Fonagy, P., & Gabbard, G. (2013). *Psychoterapia psychodynamiczna zaburzeń osobowości* [*Psychodynamic psychotherapy of personality disorders*]. Wydawnictwo Uniwersytetu Jagiellońskiego.

Czabała, Cz. (2006). *Czynniki leczące w psychoterapii* [*Therapeutic factors in psychotherapy*]. PWN.

Fairburn, C. G. (2013). *Terapia behawiorlano-poznawcza i zaburzenia odżywiania* [*Cognitive-behavioral therapy and eating disorders*]. Wydawnictwo Uniwersyetu Jagiellońskiego.

Fredrickson, B. L., & Roberts T. A. (1997). Objectification theory. Toward understanding women's lived experiences and mental health risks. *Psychology of Women Quarterly, 21*(2), 173–206. 10.1111/j.1471-6402.1997.tb00108.x

Gabbard, G. (2015). *Psychiatria psychodynamiczna w praktyce klinicznej* [Psychodynamic psychiatry in clinical practice]. Wydawnictwo Naukowe Uniwersytetu Jagiellońskiego.

Glickauf-Hughes Ch., & Wells M. (1997). *Object relations psychotherapy. An individual and integreative approach to diagnosis and treatment.* Jason Aronson, Inc.

Grzesiuk, L. (2005). (Ed.). *Psychoterapia. Teoria* [Psychotherapy. Theory]. Eneteia.

Iniewicz, G., Józefik, B., Namysłowska, I., & Ulasińska, R. (2002). Obraz relacji rodzinnych w oczach pacjentek chorujących na anoreksję psychiczną - częśc II [The subjective picture of family relations in female anorexia patients – Part II]. *Psychiatria Polska, 36*(1), 65–81.

Izydorczyk, B. (2015). *Postawy i zachowania wobec własnego ciała w zaburzeniach odżywiania* [Attitudes and behaviors towards the body in eating disorders]. PWN.

Izydorczyk, B. (2017). Psychoterapia zaburzeń obrazu ciała w anoreksji i bulimii psychicznej: podejście integracyjne (zastosowanie terapii psychodynamicznej i technik psychodramy) [Psychotherapy of body image distortions in anorexia and bulimia: An integrative approach (using elements of psychodynamic psychotherapy and psychodrama techniques)]. *Psychoterapia, 1*(180), 5–22.

Izydorczyk, B., Sitnik-Warchulska, K., Lizińczyk, S., & Lipiarz, A. (2019). Psychological predictors of unhealthy eating attitudes in young adults. *Frontiers in Psychology, 10*, 590. 10.3389/fpsyg.2019.00590

Izydorczyk, B., Sitnik-Warchulska, K., Lizińczyk, S., & Lipowska, M. (2020). Sociocultural standards promoted by the mass media as predictors of restrictive and bulimic behavior. *Frontiers in Psychiatry, 11*(506), 1–14. 10.3389/fpsyt.2020.00506

Jaworski, M., Klimkowska, K., Różańska, K., & Fabisiak, A. (2017). Rehabilitacja żywieniowa w jadłowstręcie psychicznym: rola i zakres pracy dietetyka w zespole terapeutycznym [Nutritional rehabilitation in anorexia: The role and responsibility of the dietetician in the therapeutic team]. *Medycyna Ogólna i Nauki o Zdrowiu, 23*(2), 122–128.

Józefik, B. (Ed.) (1999). *Anoreksja i bulimia psychiczna. Rozumienie i leczenie zaburzeń odżywiania się* [*Anorexia and bulimia. Understanding and treatment of eating disorders*]. Wydawnictwo Uniwersytetu Jagiellońskiego.

Józefik, B. (2014). *Kultura, ciało, (nie)jedzenie* [*Culture, body, (not)eating*]. Wydawnictwo Uniwersytetu Jagiellońskiego.

Józefik, B., Iniewicz, G., Namysłowska, I., & Ulasińska, R. (2002). Obraz relacji rodzinnych w oczach pacjentek chorujących na anoreksję psychiczną – część I [The subjective picture of family relations in female anorexia patients – Part I]. *Psychiatria Polska, 1*, 51–64.

Kernberg, O. F. (1996). A psychoanalytic theory of personality disorders. In J. F. Clarkin, & M. F. Lenzenweger (Eds.), *Major theories of personality disorders* (pp. 106–140). The Guilford Press.

Krueger, D. W. (2002a). Psychodynamic perspective on body image. In T. F. Cash, & T. Pruzinsky (Eds.), *Body image. A handbook of theory, research, and clinical practice* (pp. 30–37). The Guilford Press.

Krueger, D. W. (2002b). *Integrating body self and psychological self. Creating a new story in psychoanalysis and psychotherapy.* Bruner-Routledge.

Lewitt, A., Brzęczek, K., & Krupienicz, K. (2008). Interwencje żywieniowe w leczeniu anoreksji – wskazówki dietetyczne [Dietary interventions in treating anorexia – dietetic suggestions]. *Endokrynologia, Otyłość i Zaburzenia Przemiany Materii, 4*(3), 128–136.

Lowen, A. (2020). *Duchowość ciała. Bioenergetyka w terapii ciała i duszy* [*Spirituality and the body*]. Czarna Owca.

McWilliams, N. (2014). *Diagnoza psychoanalityczna* [*Psychoanalytic diagnosis*]. Gdańskie Wydawnictwo Psychologiczne.

Porges, S. W. (2020). *Teoria poliwagalna* [*Polyvagal theory*]. Wydawnictwo Uniwersytetu Jagiellońskiego.

Rosenberg, S. (2020). *Terapeutyczna moc nerwu błędnego. Praca z ciałem oparta na teorii poliwagalnej* [*Accessing the healing power of the vagus nerve: Self-help exercises for anxiety, depression, trauma, and autism*]. Wydawnictwo Uniwersytetu Jagiellońskiego.

Sullivan, H. S. (2001). *The interpersonal theory of psychiatry*. Routledge Taylor & Francis Group.

Summers, R. F., & Barber, J. P. (2014). *Terapia psychodynamiczna. Praktyka oparta na dowodach* [*Psychodynamic therapy: A guide to evidence-based practice*]. Wydawnictwo Uniwersytetu Jagiellońskiego.

7 Psychodrama in psychological therapy of body image distortions

This chapter presents the psychological justification for and description of the psychodrama and in the individual and group therapy, in which the protagonists are patients with eating disorders. The patients usually focus on the topics of hatred of the body and conflicts around eating. Psychodrama techniques can significantly accelerate the process of working through and/or bypassing resistance when identifying emotional and cognitive body image distortions. When the patients in psychological therapy choose the role of the in the exercises proposed by the therapist regarding body image or eating disorder symptoms, they have a chance to quickly overcome the phenomenon of universal resistance. This supports the patient's positive motivation to work on the internal causes behind body image distortions and eating disorder symptoms. Properly selected psychodrama techniques enable a quick regression in the patients, in which they can fulfill the needs that were frustrated during childhood. With the help of the auxiliary ego and role changes, the protagonist/patient can be provided with corrective emotional experiences concerning previously unmet needs.

Psychodrama and the body image in eating disorders (characteristics of basic techniques)

The organization and structure of psychodrama, along with the techniques used in the group therapy of eating disorders, are based on similar assumptions and principles as all other group therapies for patients with other neurotic and personality disorders (Bielańska, 2009). Both in individual and group therapies, various verbal and nonverbal psychodrama techniques may be used (Bielańska, 2009). By lessening resistance, they help to quickly and easily facilitate the so-called warming up, that is, internal readiness to work on emotional conflicts and deficits related to the body image. Psychodrama during group sessions in which the protagonists are patients with eating disorders usually focuses on the topics of hatred of the body, fear of sexuality, family relationships (often also conflicts with the mother), or conflicts around food and eating (Carnabucci & Ciotola, 2013). Psychodrama techniques can significantly accelerate the process of working through and/or

DOI: 10.4324/9781003251088-7

bypassing resistance when identifying emotional and cognitive body image distortions (Carnabucci & Ciotola, 2013). Exploring the body image and blocked, unconscious feelings using symbols (e.g., symbolic work with the symptoms, resistance, or obstacles) and the experience of catharsis supports the motivation to continue working on and strengthening the patient's sense of agency in patients who have hidden their feelings of weakness, helplessness, and low self-esteem in their unconscious through control and perfectionism. When the therapeutic contract is established and the patients' motivation is stabilized at a level enabling further treatment, that is, the patients made a decision to work on their internal states and symptoms, using psychodrama techniques. The therapist controls the process of warming up to psychodrama by diagnosing which patients are ready and to what extent the group (in case of group therapy) is ready to witness a psychodrama centered around the theme of unacceptable body image (Izydorczyk, 2011a, 2011b). This supports the patient's positive motivation to work on the internal causes behind body image distortions and eating disorder symptoms (Izydorczyk, 2011a, 2011b).

The technique of role changing (changing places between the protagonist and a given role, i.e., the auxiliary ego) gives the patients/protagonists an opportunity to present onstage their experiences, feelings, thoughts, and behaviors related to life history and the meaning of food and eating. Thus, they broaden the scope of knowledge about themselves and their experience of situations related, for example, to feeding, eating, the relationship with their mother, and so forth. The auxiliary ego (roles assigned by the protagonist to other group members taking part in the psychodrama) helps the protagonists become aware of the unconscious areas of their internal conflicts. "Lending voice and body" (by other patients in a group, props, or the leader/therapist in a monodrama) as well as dialog in subsequent role changes gives the opportunity not only to discover unconscious content, but also correct that which is dysfunctional (Bielańska, 2009). The patients/protagonists can hear an internal dialog with themselves on stage. By swapping roles with their stomach or other important body parts, they can become aware of their feelings toward these body parts and how much they are harming them through their behaviors, and thus activate the way to confrontation and behavior change.

The mirror technique (the patients/protagonists look at the image on the stage from the audience's perspective, from the so-called metaposition, while their place on the stage is taken by a selected double), as well as the duplication technique allow for easier and faster expression of blocked resistance (aggression) and other feelings that young patients do not see or fear experiencing/revealing.

Doubling is the "inner voice" of the protagonists spoken on their behalf by the therapist/leader from the position of the hidden "I" of the protagonist (Bielańska, 2009). It allows for expressing and venting the many hidden negative emotions experienced by the patient. They often include shame due to feeling weak and fat phobia. Doubling can have a supportive (reinforcing the protagonist's statements), confronting (provoking the protagonist to reveal feelings and thoughts), or ambivalent (showing the protagonists their contradictory feelings, thoughts, and inner conflicts) character. The leader can say what the protagonist is afraid to name outright (e.g., reveal the layers of hidden anger, and fear of adulthood, responsibility, or separation), and thus support the process of gaining insight into the psychological mechanisms underlying the eating disorder. Work with the use of the so-called phenomenon of surplus reality, often used in psychodrama, allows for corrective emotional experiences that the patients did not experience over the course of their development, for example, due to an emotionally deficient family environment (lack of satisfaction of basic needs in the family; Bielańska, 2009).

Patients with anorexia and/or bulimia function on a specific level of thinking, using body metaphors as opposed to psychological ones. For many of them, the body is not only a "hated object that needs to be controlled," but also "a constant reminder that they exist and their existence is deficient" (Levens, 2000). This "pathological deficit" forces behaviors intended to prevent the feeling of bodily fragmentation. The body, which is identified with the material object, is experienced as the "accuser," and therefore must be controlled before it "devours" the patient. Such patients have suffered a developmental failure at the stage of mental separation from the maternal object, which caused a narcissistic fixation on the body and which blocked the ability to relate to objects in the external world. A significant consequence of the failure to separate from the maternal object is the failure to develop the boundaries between the Self and the object and achieve individualization (Levens, 2000). Such a pattern of functioning is based on a profound mind–body dichotomy in which the body is perceived as an object. The patient struggles with the objectification of the body, which is often combined with a violent attack on the Self in an attempt to regain a sense of identity. The body thus becomes a scene of battle, the intensity of which stems from the fact that it does not contain only the "bad" object. In order to gain a sense of "having space" within themselves, the patients must have bodily boundaries that separate them from the world. Patients with eating disorders often struggle to cope with difficult thoughts related to the body and try to get rid of them through specific symptomatic behaviors. The more the patient tries to remove such thoughts, the more the thinking process becomes disturbed. The psychodrama stage creates a specific space for the thoughts that eating disorder patients typically want to avoid or get rid of. This provides an opportunity to employ surplus reality, both in psychodrama and in monodrama (Bielańska, 2009). Verbal and nonverbal psychodrama techniques and the assumed possibility of introducing a state of internal soothing and emotional calmness (according to Porges' polyvagal theory) provide the basis for the cognitive restructuring of the body image, and thus accelerate the cognitive and emotional insight into the psychological mechanisms of eating disorders and distortion.

In group psychotherapy (short and medium term) of eating disorders, it is worth considering the interventions supporting the transition from "eating topics" to relationships and areas beyond eating and food. Structured (also psychodramatic) exercises can be helpful in achieving this goal. For patients with bulimia and anorexia, it is important to allow themselves to be more spontaneous and creative. They feel more at ease when the therapeutic exercises are structured. As therapy progresses, it is possible to gradually abandon the structure and explore the patients' creativity and spontaneity through a psychodramatic game on stage (Izydorczyk, 2011b).

The dominant feature of patients with eating disorders is their inability to defer gratification. When a desire/need arises, there is a tendency to satisfy it immediately, and frustration demands quick discharge. The goal of psychotherapy is to teach how to delay needs gratification and tolerate the frustration. Psychodrama, for example, through surplus reality, can be used toward this goal. In the topics introduced by patients, the desire to have the so-called "good mother" often appears. This character is often identified with the therapist. Introducing the topic of the relationship with the mother onto the stage may give the patients a chance to identify and differentiate their inner feelings and states and to have corrective emotional experiences, to hear from themselves that which they wanted to, but did not hear from the mother during early childhood. In working on the insight into the psychological mechanisms of eating disorders, the patients begin assuming control over the course of the psychodrama and gain the ability to stop or slow down the pace of the work (Izydorczyk, 2011b). By analyzing the symptoms of their eating disorders, they become aware that they will not be pressured by the leader/therapist to work with areas that are currently too difficult. As subjects, they decide the pace and direction of the process.

Monodrama in the individual therapy of body image distortions

In the context of destructive thinking about oneself and one's own body image, monodrama techniques can be incorporated in individual therapy. Monodrama is a kind of psychodrama used without the participation of the group, only in the presence of the leader and the protagonist (Bielańska, 2009). The roles (the auxiliary ego) are played by props chosen by the patient/protagonist. Within monodrama, the patients work on their symptoms (especially binging and purging and the associated guilt) using the techniques of mirroring, doubling, and role changing (Bielańska, 2009).

In working on negative feelings toward one's body and oneself, it is possible to suggest expressing these feelings in a symbolic form (e.g., by representing emotions through objects of various colors). By using symbols, the patients have the opportunity to experience their emotions through tactile contact, and the therapist/leader can facilitate this exploration with questions about the details of that feeling (how strong, deep, or old it is, how is it structured, where it comes from, etc.). In turn, the patients can bypass resistance and begin to identify the feelings experienced toward themselves. On the other hand, the therapist can make an initial diagnosis of the psychological determinants of the patient's symptoms. When the patients/protagonists talk about their feelings, for example, "I'm ashamed and scared," the therapist can ask them to create an image of these emotions on stage using props as symbols. Afterwards, the patient can change roles on the stage to embody different thoughts and experiences (e.g., uncertainties related to starting treatment) which then enter into an interview with the leader/therapist. Changing roles with feelings of horror or shame, the patients/protagonists have the opportunity to symbolically (though clearly) express their sources in conversation with the therapist/leader asking exploratory questions (e.g., "How big are you?" "How old are you?" "What do you look like?"). At deeper stages of the therapeutic relationship, introducing psychodrama techniques is more effective and often allows for faster (compared to verbal dialog) warming up, that is, arousing emotions in order to facilitate sensitizing and reflection, leading to the exploration of unconscious conflicts and psychological mechanisms underlying the eating disorder symptoms.

Monodrama can be used in the initial phase of individual psychodynamic therapy when the therapeutic alliance and relationship is being built. The role of the auxiliary ego is played by props. The patients can change roles with the props and use these shifts in position to recognize selected aspects of their unconscious emotional experiences (Bielańska, 2009; Blatner, 1997; Stadler, 2018). Unlike group psychodrama, monodrama must take into account the limitations in scope and time. This also applies to the initial phase, when warming up techniques are used.

The introduction of warming up techniques to work on emotional conflicts behind body image distortions requires great care in selecting and adapting them to safe contact with the body. In patients who treat the body as an unacceptable "bad object" that must be destroyed, contact with the body through touch should be introduced gradually and carefully (both in group and individual therapy). Introducing such exercises too quickly may be traumatizing for such patients, especially if they experienced abuse/ violation of boundaries before.

The use of psychodrama in facilitating insight in eating disorders

Insight is also important in psychodrama. The protagonists/patients with eating disorders recreates their internal conflicts with the help of the auxiliary ego (actors or props), also in order to gain insight into their unconscious motives, emotions, conflicts, and so forth (Izydorczyk, 2011b). Intellectual reflection on their inner world presented onstage often becomes a source of insight. This is due to the possibility of seeing the psychodramatic scene, which the patients have created themselves, "from the sidelines." Group members in the auxiliary ego role, for example, playing the role of symptoms such as a distorted body image or binge eating and purging behaviors, as well as various body parts and organs (the stomach after purging) may show the protagonist what is taking place, thus emphasizing the cognitive aspects of the mechanisms of eating disorders (Izydorczyk, 2011b). The protagonists/patients can recognize and experience their own emotions related to the body, food, eating, and eating disorder symptoms by assuming the role of their body parts or organs that are "tormented" by the symptoms and self-destructive behaviors. They experience a part of themselves and have the opportunity to deepen the emotional insight into the symbolic meaning and development of eating disorder symptoms (Izydorczyk, 2009).

Apart from supporting the patient's insight, an important therapeutic factor in psychodrama involves the possibility of corrective emotional experiences through surplus reality. This means giving the patients/protagonists the opportunity to experience onstage those emotions/needs that were absent in their development. This often significantly repairs the patient's emotional deficits or unmet needs and the resulting developmental deficits. As mentioned previously, the symptomatology of eating disorders is often based on disorders in the personality structure. Therefore, including both insight and corrective actions (dialog and the therapeutic relationship supported by elements of mono- and psychodrama within psychodynamic therapy) is warranted.

Psychodrama provides the patients with many constructive solutions: the leader becomes an important adult who usually (if selected to take part in mono- or psychodrama in group therapy) is endowed with special trust, eliminating of guilt and shame. In a way, they assume the role of the "good enough mother." Psychodrama teaches not to feel fear, shame, or guilt because it gives the opportunity to act out various difficult emotions on stage and experience catharsis, treating the drama as an externalized element of reality.

Properly selected psychodrama techniques enable a quick regression in the patients/protagonists, in which they can fulfill the needs that were frustrated during childhood. With the help of the auxiliary ego and role changes, the protagonists/patients can be provided with corrective emotional experiences concerning previously unmet needs (Izydorczyk, 2009, 2011b). Through the technique of doubling and role changing, they also gain the possibility of insight into the unconscious phenomena of their inner emotional world. Finally, working with surplus reality provides a chance to correct past frustrations due to a lack of an appropriate "maternal environment." Regression and surplus reality techniques are important therapeutic factors. During psychodrama, previously unconscious internal conflicts are externalized, which allows them to be significantly modified and transformed. In working with patients with eating disorders, great emphasis is placed on the relationship between the patients' body, thoughts, and emotions related to their physicality. As many memories stored in the body reach the preverbal level, paying attention to the patients' interoceptive signals allows for expanding their bodily awareness. The etiology of eating disorders includes the failure of the mother to adequately identify and respond to the child's somatic signals (see Chapter 5). The use of psychodrama techniques (e.g., role changing) may be helpful in exploring this matrix of relationships with a significant object as well as with its internal representation. This improves insight into unconscious emotions and mechanisms of disorders in a sick person. The patients/protagonists changing roles with their mother provides an opportunity to experience the ambivalent feelings toward her.

A face-to-face meeting is one of the positions of therapeutic work often subject to modifications in various modalities, for example, psychoanalytical and psychodynamic psychotherapy and psychodrama. There is a very active meeting between the therapist and the eating disorder patient, where the patient, playing out his inner drama, shows it to the therapist and the group. The therapists/leaders, unlike a typical analyst, do not provide interpretations onstage, but rather join the drama: they are involved on the stage, are transparent, and support the patient's (and the group's) spontaneity. In psychodrama, actions performed directly on stage dominate, inviting discharge of emotions related to outside situations (acting in). The patients/ protagonists playing out their inner experiences (conflicts, emotions) on stage have a chance to experience catharsis, support the process of compensating for their deficits, and thus improve poorly integrated personality structures (Bielańska, 2009).

Psychodrama focuses on the present, although the role of the past in the patient's life is not denied. The past is often played out onstage in the here and now, which allows past conflicts to be relived, for example, by surplus reality. Working on the topic of deficits in the relationship with the parents or other significant objects in the past, the patients have the opportunity to experience the psychodrama process in the here and now, and gain insight into the source of their symptoms, self-harm behaviors, and difficulties (Izydorczyk, 2009, 2011b). It becomes possible to analyze the cause–effect relationships between the internal representation of the relationship with the significant object and the patient's current relationships.

Increasingly often, psychodrama takes into account the role and strength of recurring early childhood activities based on the relationship with significant objects. On the one hand, psychodrama emphasizes the necessity of the protagonists' free choice on the stage (they create their reality contained there and they decide how to act within it). On the other hand, increasingly often the patients allow their past to be brought onto the stage in the here and now. The concept of time has a specific character in psychodrama. The corrective, therapeutic actions cover the past, present, and future (including confrontations with unwanted or undesirable situations, events, or outcomes). The events onstage, focusing on the patient's problems, as well as the patient/protagonist assuming the roles of his body parts or organs, hearing specific, often unwanted (unconscious) voices, and experiencing impulses or emotions, allow for the unconscious, unwanted, and difficult mental and emotional content to be made conscious and accepted much more effectively (Izydorczyk, 2011b). Taking the position of a mirror (standing on the side, the metaposition) gives the patients the possibility of cognitive insight into their inner and outer worlds. On the other hand, role changes allow for hearing the most hidden content from the double, while using surplus reality gives the opportunity for emotional insight, catharsis, and corrective emotional experiences.

Psychodramatic work on internalized early childhood relationships can become significant because the patient/protagonist has the possibility of correcting them through the use of surplus reality. Due to acting in, the inner world of the protagonist is transferred to the stage in the psychodramatic game. The auxiliary ego behaves as the protagonist imagines, meaning that it is based on transference. Often, the protagonist carries the theme of the group, recreating transference patterns which can be corrected (the projections can be removed) through the psychodrama. The patient may transfer the function of the parent to the leader (similarly to the analytical or psychodynamic therapist). In psychodrama, transference can even be given a role, provoked, and resolved. Transference can be resolved mainly through dismissal from the role and *sharing* (after the protagonists' psychodrama ends, each group member "takes" a subject or theme they shared with the group back into their own internal experience).

Work on transference should not be limited to an extensive psychodrama or a smaller vignette (a single scene depicting a selected internal aspect of the patient, without role changes), but it should also be elaborated during individual of group sessions of psychodynamic therapy. When the patients working on their relationship with another group member or the therapist, based on experiencing inadequate aggression, experience the need to discharge this aggression (catharsis), treating it as an element of the psychodrama "without leaving the chair" encourages visualization and expression together with a simultaneous analysis of the transference themes at the source of the aggression. For patients with eating disorders who are competing for attention for their symptoms with other group members with similar diagnoses, the empty chair technique may help better recognize the transference of the maternal relationship by the patient onto other group members who identify with them (Izydorczyk, 2009). The therapists, standing behind the patient's chair, may also intensify this process by using duplication, that is, expressing themselves what is difficult for the patient to express. It is worth taking into account the fact that patients with eating disorders develop different personality structure psychopathologies, from the neurotic to the psychotic. Due to this, both psychodynamic and psychodrama works require an individualized approach to patient resistance.

Psychodrama techniques allow for working on resistance in, for example, group psychotherapy. Here, the thematically selected group games (anti-social family, tiger fights, joint expedition) are used to work on the so-called cleaning (explaining) of relations between group members, along with sociometric techniques and duplication. In psychodrama, resistance appears during so-called "difficult scenes" which arouse feelings of shame in the patient/protagonist. In patients with eating disorders, the mini-dramas played on stage often concern precisely the topics that evoke shame, fear, and withdrawal: body image (often associated with disgust) and eating disorder symptoms. As a significant object, using appropriate interventions (similarly to a psychodynamic therapist), the leader/therapist removes the responsibility for these feelings from the protagonist/patient, with the difference being that they are expressed onstage and thus reduced or removed.

Psychodrama and the body image in anorexia

In the next stage of treatment, when the patient with anorexia has established a therapeutic relationship with the therapist, there is a time to work with the symptoms, internal conflicts, and internalized relationships with significant objects in order to correct developmental deficits. In both group and individual therapies, it is also possible to use various psychodrama techniques. They facilitate quicker warming up, that is, the internal readiness to work on emotional conflicts and deficits. When the patients in group therapy choose a role in the warming up phase (e.g., in psychodramatic games on the topic of a trip together), they can observe other patients in the group playing their roles, listen to the analysis and discussion in the final phase, get feedback from others as well as share their own experiences with others. This helps quickly overcome universal resistance and motivate the patients to work on the internal causes of their eating disorder symptoms (Bielańska, 2009; Izydorczyk, 2009, 2011b). At this stage, it is worth considering the elements of visualization (imagining the body image as a whole or in various parts), psychodrawing (e.g., making a body map), and dance (especially in group work), through which patients with anorexia learn to contact their own body in a noninvasive way. An example can be a group dance in a circle, during which the participants do not hold hands, but hold a string connecting them (a symbol of communication). They are able to maintain a distance that is appropriate for them at this stage and which protects from excessive (threatening) physical closeness.

Adolescents are often diagnosed with anorexia. As it results from the specificity of this developmental period and the identity crisis it involves, they experience adolescent rebellion indirectly, through disease symptoms. Such patients usually take part in group therapy. Through psychodramatic games and the roles they assume, they can learn to recognize the psychological mechanisms and internal conflicts behind eating disorder symptoms (e.g., fear of responsibility, adult life, or intimacy, acceptance of own sexuality) in a noninvasive way (bypassing resistance). They can also experience catharsis in supportive conditions (a group of people experiencing similar issues). In psychodrama, this means not only unblocking and expressing negative emotions, but also being filled with positive emotions, often through surplus reality. It means the possibility of acting on the stage where the protagonist's reality differs from the actual reality of the patient (Bielańska, 2009).

In psychodramatic work on the symptom of restrictive weight loss and the search for its psychological sources, the dominant techniques are role changing, role training, doubling, mirroring, and working with surplus reality.

Role changing (i.e., the protagonist taking the role of the auxiliary ego) gives the patients/protagonists a chance to show onstage their experiences related to life, food and eating, and individual body parts, as well as specific feelings, thoughts, and behaviors. Through this, they broaden the scope of knowledge about themselves and their experiences. The auxiliary ego helps the protagonist/patient to become aware of unconscious conflicts because by "lending a voice and body" (by another person in a group, a prop, or the leader/therapist in a monodrama) and by dialog in subsequent role changes, it makes it possible not only to discover the unconscious, but also to correct the dysfunctional. The patients/protagonists can hear an internal dialog with themselves on the stage. As already mentioned, in switching roles with their stomach or other important body part, they can become aware of the feelings and (self-destructive) behaviors toward them, and thus activate the way to confrontation and change.

The mirror technique (the patients/protagonists look at the onstage situation "from the side," the metaposition, while their place on stage is taken by the chosen double) as well as the duplication technique allow for easier and faster therapy, revealing blocked rebellion (aggression) and other feelings that the patient does not notice or fears expressing. Doubling (having the protagonists' "inner voice" spoken on their behalf by the therapist/leader from the position of the protagonist's hidden "I") also allows to relieve fat phobia and unconscious negative emotions (e.g., shame, aversion, or anger) toward the body.

Psychodrama with patients with anorexia is often combined with art therapy as represented by Lacey and Evans (1986). It is tied to the psychoanalytical theory and object relations theory. It assumes that the expression of unconscious thoughts and feelings is mostly done with images, not words. Similar assumptions can be found in Porges' (2020) polyvagal theory and its recommendations for vagus nerve stimulation and preverbal techniques in bodywork (Carnabucci & Ciotola, 2013; Rosenberg, 2020). Art therapy techniques (music therapy and choreotherapy, including psychodrama) allow the use of an alternative, preverbal language in working with resistance, bypassing the patient's defense mechanisms (usually the repressed aspect of the self can be expressed more freely through an image, because words are easier to control). Regarding therapy of anorexia, Levens (2000) draws attention to the importance of the patients' relationship to their own body, thoughts, and emotions. Many memories stored in the body reach the preverbal level, hence, paying attention to the patients' interoceptive signals enables them to expand their body awareness. Psychodrama grants many opportunities to overcome defenses and anxiety, to identify and name feelings, thoughts, and needs, as well as to gain emotional and intellectual insight into the psychological mechanisms behind anorexic symptoms and body image distortions.

The use of psychodrama techniques in working on body image in bulimia

In patients with bulimia, low self-esteem determines negative (self-destructive) thinking about oneself and the world ("I am nobody, nothing"). When patients with bulimia seek treatment, they often show initial motivation to get rid of bothersome (embarrassing, guilty, even disgusting) binge eating and/or purging behaviors. When there is time to build a therapeutic alliance and establish the contract, psychodrama techniques such as role changing or the mirror technique are often included in the verbal dialog with the patient. The scene is not only a physical space where the psychodramatic image of the protagonists'/patients' life can be portrayed, but is also a symbolic presentation of the patients' inner world, for example, the feelings they experience in connection with beginning treatment (Izydorczyk, 2009, 2011b).

In the first stage of individual contact with the patient, the therapist can suggest work with imagery and visualization techniques. Sometimes, if the patients respond to the suggestion to go on stage with resistance (they are silent or categorically refuse), it is worth working on the sources of their resistance using therapeutic dialog, and then to propose image construction without having the patients leave their chair. An example includes showing onstage (in front of the patients' chair) what prevents them from making a decision about treatment or what prevented them from seeking help earlier. An important element of therapy is the introduction of the auxiliary ego in the form of symbolic roles (props chosen by the patients, symbolically representing parts of the image they create). Using these objects, a resisting, silent, impulsive, or self-hating patients can indicate what they see or feel without having to evaluate what they are doing. Through an interview with the patient/protagonist done before the psychodrama, while the patient is still arranging the props in front of him to reflect his experience, the therapist/leader can initiate a so-called continuation, aimed at exploring the motivation for treatment and/or the source of the patient's symptoms (what blocked feelings or internal conflicts lay behind the symptoms). When the patients' activity increases (they respond to questions, choose props, and arrange them according to their own internal image of what they see and feel), it is possible to propose to get up from the chair and play out the images on stage. The therapist analyzes how the patients' expressed state came about, why they resisted the psychodrama previously, what obstacles they encountered on their way to decide on therapy, what feelings are dominating, and what they see in their inner world regarding their symptoms and body image. Working on emotions with the use of symbols is justified here.

Both the author's clinical experience as well as the literature on the subject show that patients (especially women) with bulimia often raise the topic of negative (self-destructive) feelings directed toward their bodies. The dominant ones among them are disgust, shame, anger, fear, and self-destructive impulses (Józefik, 1999; Lacey & Evans, 1986). If the patients signal disgust toward themselves or their body in relation to binge eating and purging, it is good to suggest that they show this disgust in a symbolic form (e.g., the patients choose an object from a colored set to symbolize their disgust). By symbolizing disgust with a prop, the patient has the opportunity to perceive and experience it, and the therapist can ask about the specific features of this feeling (how big, strong, deep, old it is, what structure does it have, where does it come from, etc.). The patients, in turn, have the opportunity to bypass resistance and thus make a preliminary identification of the feeling they experience toward themselves and the therapist – a preliminary identification of the psychological determinants of their symptoms. When the patients/protagonists talk about their feelings (e.g., "I'm ashamed and terrified"), the therapist can suggest to arrange a picture of their emotions onstage (demonstrate the feelings using symbolic props). After building this picture, the therapist can ask the patient to change roles, that is, assume the role of a given part of the picture. From the changed role, the patients/protagonists can show (with the help of the therapist/leader's exploring questions) their thinking and experiencing of various aspects of themselves (e.g., the ambivalence about treatment).

Revealing self-destructive feelings onstage by the patient and communicating understanding and acceptance by the therapist encourages the patient to be more spontaneous and to counter the pathological impulsivity of the bulimic symptoms of binge eating and purging. By asking questions in the psychodramatic interview, the therapist/leader can indicate the negative aspects of the feelings that the patient is not consciously aware of while showing support and readiness to accompany the patient in difficult decisions related to treatment and daily coping with self-destructive symptoms and feelings (especially guilt). From the position of the mirror, the patients/protagonists can look at the image onstage from the side while their place is taken by the chosen double. By taking the observer position and avoiding an overly emotional attitude, the patients can gain cognitive insight into the sources of bulimic symptoms as they are portrayed on stage.

The specificity of psychodrama in working on a symptom (case study)

Once the therapeutic relationship has been established, the patients usually begin to slowly discover how difficult it is for them to bear their symptoms and how reluctant they are to acknowledge that bulimia involves relapses that must be accounted for. In patients with bulimia, low self-esteem determines negative (self-destructive) thinking about oneself and the world ("I am nobody, nothing").

Warm-up phase

In one of the weekly sessions in the fourth month of individual psychodynamic therapy, the bulimic patient began by discussing what happened between sessions: the shame and guilt that she experienced during a cycle of binge eating and purging two days prior. Sitting in the chair, she said that she still felt that "something was gripping her," that her stomach ached, and that she had no respect for her body. When asked what she meant by "something gripping her," she replied that may be it was the feelings she was talking about, but she did not understand them. The patient indicated directly how difficult it was for her to reveal the actions for which she blames herself and her feelings of shame and anxiety. As the patient spoke of disrespect to her body, she was holding her stomach. She was asked to pay attention to this fact and to describe what she felt now. She focused on this part of her body because it was where she focused her attention and touch. Through direct contact with the body, she could feel her stomach. For the therapist, the patient's contact with the sensations flowing from her stomach was a specific phase of the patient's warming up to continue working on her bulimic symptoms (binge eating and purging). Further in the session, the patient was invited to work on the symptoms using imagery onstage. The therapist asked the patient what she felt when she touched her stomach, to which she replied that she was still experiencing guilt, anger, and shame. These emotions were built up on the stage.

Scene I. Building the image of the patient's feelings: "Guilt, anger, and shame"

The therapist suggested that the patient should lay out the feelings she was feeling now in front of her, marking them with colored scarves of her choice. The patient picked a red scarf for shame, a black one for anger, and a gray one for guilt. When asked for the title of this scene, she replied that she could not name it directly. However, by making a symbolic choice of the scarves for the roles of shame, anger, and guilt, she was already conveying something unconscious. The red color of shame could suggest the intensity and ambivalence of this emotion. This color symbolizes intensity, and on the other hand, vitality (the color of blood). Maybe this intensity could be targeted further? The black scarf chosen for the role of anger could symbolize depression, helplessness, and aggression. The gray scarf of guilt symbolized suppression, helplessness, and ambiguity. When the patient built her own image, she refused to change roles with any of the feelings onstage.

The therapist decided it was too early for confrontations. The therapist stated that at this stage of her work, the patient is not "emotionally warmed up" and needs more time. The therapist then used the mirror technique – introduced a prop (a white scarf chosen by the patient), which assumed the role of the auxiliary ego (i.e., the double) and placed it in a spot indicated by the patient (between shame, anger, and guilt). From the observer's position, the patient saw the image of her feelings and commented "this is my interior: guilt, anger, shame." This was how she directly named her inner states.

In sharing feedback, the patient talked about the feeling guilt and shame because of her symptoms ("I am ashamed of my symptoms, this feeling has been with me throughout my whole life"). As the session was ending, the therapist strengthened the patient's resources, released her from feeling guilty for the symptoms, and supported her courage in facing such a difficult topic. The therapist "allowed" the patient to experience shame as something that exists and is permissible (Izydorczyk, 2009).

During the next several sessions, the patient reported an improvement in mental well-being (lower depression, shame, and guilt after binge eating and purging), but she still complained of persistent bulimic cycles occurring with a frequency of 2–3 times per day. In one of the next sessions, she said at the beginning, holding her stomach, "I'm fed up with this, I gorged myself again and vomited, now everything hurts and my stomach burns." The therapist asked her to focus on what she feels when touching her stomach (and closing her eyes to strengthen the interoceptive sensations). The patient, with her eyes closed, kept her hand on her stomach for a moment in silence. Without opening her eyes, she said, "I hear my stomach gurgling, I feel something ache in my stomach, now I feel like telling it that I am disgusting for doing this to it, but I can't stop." The therapist asked the patient to open her eyes and suggested a monodrama on stage. The monodrama entitled "Belly" was conducted onstage, with the patient selecting a symbol for her stomach. The therapist proposed changing roles with the stomach and conducted a psychodramatic interview in such a way that the patient could feel and see what sensations her stomach experiences in a situation when she torments it with binge eating and purging. In this way, she was able to better experience the ambivalence of the pain and suffering of her stomach rather than just the relief from vomiting, which she often talked about in earlier sessions.

The patient, playing the role of the stomach, signaled that she had lost control over the binge eating and purging ("I don't know why I'm doing this, I have some form of anxiety"). The therapist then asked what is bothering the patient and the stomach more – the anxiety or the vomiting. The patient in the role of the stomach replied: "I will bear it, it will pass." The therapist then asked the patient in the role of the stomach how it helps her cope with her anxiety. The patient/stomach revealed her feelings. The therapist then asked: "What unsettled matters do you have?" The patient replied: "I have to take a look at what happened 4 years ago, it is unfinished, that was the period I started overeating." Reflecting afterwards, the patient indicated her readiness to meet onstage with her binge eating and purging in the near future, after which another monodrama was scheduled and the session was finished (Izydorczyk, 2009).

At an advanced stage of the therapeutic process, when the bulimic patient has established a therapeutic relationship, there is time to work with the symptoms, internal conflicts, and internalized relations with significant objects in order to correct developmental deficits. Individual psychodynamic therapy of the patient presented above included insight-oriented work on internal conflicts, the diagnosis and changing of pathological coping mechanisms, and interpretation of transference. Monodramas focused on the use of the symbolic plane in working with the bulimic symptoms, the resulting guilt, as well as the increasing emotional tension and self-disgust. This gave the therapist the opportunity to reveal emotional conflicts and the specific ways of experiencing them onstage, and contributed to the exploration of accumulated tension and emotions (especially negative ones) which the patient unconsciously "released" through the symptoms. Work onstage "loosens" the controlling function and the "constant readiness to act in defense" of the patient's psychological mechanisms.

At an advanced stage of the above patient's individual therapy, the monodrama contributed to provoking "internal cleansing" and relieving of tension (catharsis). Thus, a safe, more controlled decrease in emotional tension lowered the number of self-destructive symptoms. The patient's actions based on interoceptive sensations, intuition, feelings, adaptive cognitive schema, and imagination have been strengthened.

Further in treatment, with the patient's consent, the therapist suggested the patient "meet with the vomiting" so that she could consider alternative ways of coping with this symptom. Through this intervention at this stage of treatment, the therapist was slowly heading toward teaching the patient alternative ways to cope with self-destructive feelings (by allowing the patient to feel emotional ambivalence toward the symptom of vomiting). Playing out the image on the psychodrama scene shortly after an episode of binge eating and purging (as was the case with this patient), allows to analyze the episode step by step, identifying the warning signals, and offering alternative coping strategies for future episodes (Izydorczyk, 2009). By changing roles with individual aspects of the situation leading to the episode (different feelings, situational stress, interpersonal conflicts) as well as the feelings and symptoms (binge eating and vomiting), the patient can expand insight of previously unconscious aspects. This can deepen the motivation to take appropriate control over drives, impulses, feelings, and needs, while becoming aware of the destructive character of the control that patients attempt to take over their body through eating disorder symptoms.

In the initial phase of group psychodynamic therapy with patients who are heterogeneous in terms of gender and diagnosis (neurotic disorders and personality disorders), the first sessions are usually focused on building the contract (demanding confidentiality and attendance at all sessions) and the therapeutic alliance. This allows for setting boundaries and strengthens the patients' sense of security. Patients with bulimia often adopt a specific attitude in this phase: they seek guidance, structure, and immediate relief of emotional discomfort (impulsivity, shame, guilt for symptoms). The dominant and recurring theme is the relationship with the mother and the need to have a "good mother," which is often projected onto the therapist. At an advanced stage of treatment, when working on insight into the psychological mechanisms of bulimia, the patients often focus their attention on themselves, mainly introducing difficulties and problems that are thematically focused on eating and bulimic symptoms. They pay less attention to other group members and they reveal guilt in their comments. The peculiarity of their process is that after their own psychodrama work on topics related to bulimia, they often experience increased guilt for "taking up time by focusing on themselves." In this way, they repeat the bulimic obsessive–compulsive cycle: binge eating – purging – guilt.

However, in the initial stage of group therapy, difficulties related to the area of eating is an important point in identifying and determining the group members' level of trust toward each other. It is highly therapeutic for the patients to realize in this phase of the process that other patients with bulimia also often try to hide their symptoms. Patients with bulimia often spend their energy pleasing others. The therapy group can help access the repressed, "needy" part of themselves by playing the roles that the patient/protagonist chooses, for example, "loving sister," "loyal friend," or "conscientious student." The group helps to recognize the aspects that the patient accepts in themselves, creating a comprehensive image of themselves, standing in opposition to the "bad" bulimic aspect (Jay, 2000).

The group needs help to progress to topics beyond the area of food and eating. Structured exercises can help achieve this goal. For example, the therapist might say "Let's put food aside for a moment and think about two feelings we often experience. Become these feelings and introduce yourself your partner." This exercise allows to establish a deeper identification between the members (Levens, 2000). For patients with bulimia, allowing themselves to be spontaneous is an expression of irresponsibility and recklessness, which causes guilt. Because of this they improve their self-esteem or increase confidence (Jay, 2000; Lacey & Evans, 1986). The group relaxes more when the exercises are structured. As therapy progresses, it is possible to gradually abandon the structure as of the group's tolerance increases. Before the patients feel accepted by each other in the group, they need to play out certain aspects of bulimic behaviors in the psychodrama, which often involves working with symbols, for example, a fridge or a favorite food that is consumed during binge eating episodes. Understanding the context in which the symbol is used helps uncover problem areas in the relationship sphere. The role changing technique helps in this process. The patients can meet their despair, emptiness, denied needs, and suppressed anger.

In summary, psychodrama helps patients turn abstract statements more concrete. It reduces the feeling of confusion and ambiguity, which is the main reason for the patients' problems with coping with "inner experience" and with the outside world.

Creativity and spontaneity contained in the possibilities of psychodrama can be an important element in generating cognitive and emotional insight, an inspiring source of knowledge about the patients, as well as a source of corrective emotional experiences. The integrative use of both activities in group and individual psychotherapy of patients with eating disorders may indicate a good (pro-health) prognosis for their entire treatment process.

References

Bielańska, A. (2009). *Psychodrama. Elementy teorii i praktyki* [*Psychodrama. Elements of theory and practice*]. Eneteia.

Blatner, A. (1997). Psychodrama: The state of the art. *The Arts in Psychotherapy*, *24*(1), 23–30. 10.1016/S0197-4556(96)00057-3

Carnabucci, K., & Ciotola, L. (2013). *Healing eating disorders with psychodrama and other action methods. Beyond the silence and the fury*. Jessica Kingsley Publishers.

Izydorczyk B. (2009). Psychodrama w leczeniu anoreksji psychicznej [Psychodrama in the treatment of anorexia]. In A. Bielańska (Ed.), *Psychodrama. Elementy teorii i praktyki* [*Psychodrama. Elements of theory and practice*] (pp. 267–304). Eneteia.

Izydorczyk, B. (2011a). A psychological profile of the bodily self characteristics in women suffering from bulimia nervosa. In P. Hay (Ed.), *New insights into the prevention and treatment of bulimia nervosa* (pp. 147–167). Intech Open Access Publisher.

Izydorczyk, B. (2011b). Zastosowanie psychodramy w psychoterapii pacjentów chorujących na anoreksję i bulimię psychiczną [Psychodrama in the treatment of anorexia and bulimia]. *Psychiatria Polska*, *45*(2), 261–275.

Jay S. (2000). The use of psychodrama in the field of bulimia. In D. Dokter (Ed.), *fragile board: Arts therapies and clients with eating disorders* (pp. 177–189). Jessica Kingsley Publishers.

Józefik, B. (Ed.) (1999). *Anoreksja i bulimia psychiczna. Rozumienie i leczenie zaburzeń odżywiania się* [*Anorexia and bulimia. Understanding and treatment of eating disorders*]. Wydawnictwo Uniwersytetu Jagiellońskiego.

Lacey, J. H., & Evans, C. D. H. (1986). The impulsivist: A multi-impulsive personality disorder. *British Journal of Addiction*, *81*(5), 641–649. 10.1111/j.1360-0443.1986.tb00382.x

Levens, M. (2000). Art therapy and psychodrama with eating disordered patients. In D. Dokter (Ed.). *Fragile boards. Arts therapies and clients with eating disorder* (pp. 159–176). Jessica Kingsley Publishers.

Porges, S. W. (2020). *Teoria poliwagalna* [*Polyvagal theory*]. Wydawnictwo Uniwersytetu Jagiellońskiego.

Rosenberg, S. (2020). *Terapeutyczna moc nerwu błędnego. Praca z ciałem oparta na teorii poliwagalnej* [*Accessing the healing power of the vagus nerve: Self-help exercises for anxiety, depression, trauma, and autism*]. Wydawnictwo Uniwersytetu Jagiellońskiego.

Stadler, C. (2018). *Psychodrama w teorii i praktyce* [*Psychodrama in theory and practice*]. Eneteia.

8 Summary: directions and areas of studying the diagnosis and treatment of body image distortions in eating disorders

Summarizing the data presented in this book, together with the conclusions of the analysis of theoretical and empirical literature (including the author's own studies), and keeping in mind their limitations, it is worth highlighting the fact that recognizing the psychosocial risk factors for the development of anti-health behaviors toward the body and the psychological diagnosis of disturbances in bodily experience among eating disorder (anorexia, bulimia, and binge eating disorder) is a complex and multi-stage process. From the beginning of the process, an accurate diagnosis helps to recognize and differentiate individual and discrete emotional and cognitive body image distortions in patients who do not yet exhibit typical eating disorder symptoms, but who are in a high-risk group for their development.

Psychological diagnosis requires combining psychological and medical knowledge to adjust the diagnostic process and the planning of treatment (especially psychotherapy) to the current health capabilities of the eating disorder patient. Due to its importance for the recovery process of patients exhibiting body image distortions and anti-health behaviors toward the body, it is worth to introduce complex psychological diagnosis of the characteristics of the clinical indices of body image from the moment that eating disorder symptoms appear.

Table 8.1 presents a proposed list of basic factors and their indicators important in the process of conducting a psychological diagnosis of body image distortions in patients with eating disorders.

Confirming the scientific validity of psychological diagnosis carried out in treatment of eating disorders requires (in accordance with the principles of evidence-based medical and psychological practice; American Psychological Association, 2006) systematic studies on various population samples in order to test the hypotheses concerning the emotional, cognitive, and sociocultural predictors of body image distortions and the resulting anti-health behaviors toward the body.

The basic areas of future studies should first focus on exploring the multifactorial structure of the body image (rather than merely measuring dissatisfaction with the body and its individual parts) together with measuring body esteem, the spectrum of emotions felt toward the body, the self-assessment of bodily health and fitness, behaviors related to the body, and fat phobia.

DOI: 10.4324/9781003251088-8

Table. 8.1 Clinical psychological diagnosis of psychosocial factors in body image
disorders in patients suffering from eating disorders

Psychosocial factors	Clinical diagnostic indicators
The pattern of early childhood bonds and past psychological traumas	Clinically confirmed insecure, that is, anxious, anxious–avoidant, or disorganized attachment style, emotional neglect (chronic traumatic events related to deficits in parental care and exposure to life or health risks, e.g., separation from the caregiver as a result of departure or hospitalization, lack of systematic protection, neglect, physical violence, cold or emotionally unstable parental behavior), and/or mental trauma related to the body – physical and sexual violence (excessive, restrictive parental control and interference through corporal punishment or sexual abuse).
Parental attitudes toward the body and nutrition	Analysis of transgenerational messages and family myths about the body and nutrition, eating habits, and the function of eating in the family system.
Patterns of functioning of the family system (especially the attitudes toward the children's separation and individuation) centered around fear of separation and relationships that hinder autonomy (especially in adolescents)	The description of the emotional bond between the child and the parent (caregiver) reveals excessive closeness, entanglement, overprotection, stiffness, inability to resolve conflicts, and involving the child in various marital conflicts. The family system reinforces denial of problems and incompatibilities as well as avoidance of expressing dissenting opinions and resolving conflicts. When diagnosing patients with bulimia, it is worth taking into account the presence of chaos in the family system and the important role of family conflicts, low self-esteem and childhood obesity, high expectations by the parents toward the children, and frequent critical comments about body weight and eating habits. The relationship between the parents is often based on domination and submission. Anger, mutual rejection, and blame dominate the family communication. The patient perceives their parents (especially the father) as overly focused on appearance and eating, intrusive, impulsive, and unable to meet the patient's needs. When diagnosing patients with anorexia, it is important to examine the family patterns of emotional distance in relationships, pressure, excessive criticism toward oneself, stiffness, conflict avoidance, difficulties in showing empathy, and disturbed communication (especially in the relationship with the mother) characterized by negative emotions, blame, and misunderstandings.

(Continued)

Table. 8.1 (Continued)

Psychosocial factors	Clinical diagnostic indicators
The parents' mental and psychosomatic disorders	Eating disorders, affective disorders, alcohol and substance use disorders, or other disorders in one or both parents.
Psychodynamic diagnosis of the personality structure and psychological profile	1. Clinical assessment of the resources and dynamics of the personality structure (the maturity of the ego, i.e., the level of identity integration and the ability to test reality – adequacy in the perception of the world and the Self).
	2. Assessment of the strength of defense mechanisms, especially splitting, denial, projective identification, omnipotent control, and primitive idealization.
	3. Assessment of fat phobia (obsessive concentration on food in thoughts, emotions, and behaviors, which masks conflicts related to separation and individuation).
	4. Assessment of the profile of psychological features (perfectionism, impulsivity, fear of gaining weight, fear of adulthood – especially in adolescents and young adults).
	5. Assessment of the pattern of establishing relationships (level of distrust and uncertainty).
Body image	1. Assessment of body image distortions (the level of cognitive and emotional distortions: body dissatisfaction, including the discrepancy between the real and ideal body image, dissatisfaction with general appearance and individual body parts, care for appearance and physical fitness, sense of and care for health, deficits in interoceptive awareness).
	2. Assessment of the ability to adequately perceive and feel bodily boundaries.
	3. Assessment of the frequency and character of self-destructive (restrictive and compulsive) behaviors toward the body and eating.
The influence of sociocultural factors on body image	Assessment of the level of pressure from and internalization of sociocultural body image standards as factors in regulating self-esteem.
Triggers	Assessment of particularly stressful situations in the past which contributed to the development of restrictive eating as a solution to emotional difficulties, for example, critical remarks on overweight and appearance, identifying with models, actresses, and other "successful people," using various diets (both by the patients and by their family members), religious and spiritual beliefs (an ascetic attitude toward

(*Continued*)

Table. 8.1 (Continued)

Psychosocial factors	Clinical diagnostic indicators
	renouncing pleasure), situations of changes in adolescence (changing schools, places of residence, departures, illnesses, deaths in the family), experiences of devaluation and rejection by peers, and so forth.
Supporting factors (intrapsychic and interpersonal)	Assessment of feelings of satisfaction, control, and success associated with positive comments from the environment, for example, due to weight loss, a sense of uniqueness and originality strengthening the sense of identity. At the interpersonal level (including the family), assessment of the person gaining a central position (care, importance, attention) in the family due to eating disorder symptoms, gaining privileges, lessened requirements in school, winning a peer competition in terms of body appearance.

Source: Own elaboration.

Second, future studies on body image in eating disorders should be expanded by deepening the psychological (clinical and psychometric, test-based) measurement of personality traits and structures. Patients with eating disorders often display disorders in the personality structure, and studying them would allow for understanding the specificity of emotional, cognitive, and social functioning of such patients – which coping strategies they employ in difficult every day and crisis situations as well as the psychological and biological sources of the emotional/cognitive difficulties in experiencing their corporeality and the anti-health behaviors toward the body. In the process of clinical diagnosis and testing of hypotheses related to body image among eating disorder patients, it is worth to include not only the elements of psychodynamic diagnosis based on Kernberg's structured interview, presented in this book, but also the measurement of the personality organization using the psychodynamic diagnostic model PDM 2 (Lingiardi & McWilliams, 2019). This will allow for creating a complex clinical and quantifiable description of the psychological functioning and the dynamics of the patient's personality structure. Identifying specific personality traits and structures, adaptive and defense mechanisms, unconscious internal conflicts, emotional difficulties, and patterns of establishing relationships becomes a significant element facilitating the effectiveness of the planned treatment, especially with regard to the indications for planned psychotherapy (e.g., establishing the validity of beginning psychodynamic, cognitive–behavioral, short- and long-term, individual or group therapy).

The PDM 2 diagnostic model allows for understanding the patients' psychological mechanisms of functioning, especially in terms of their internal experiences and the patterns of interpersonal relationships. It also helps to establish which therapeutic interventions are the most appropriate for a given patient. Different personality structures among eating disorder patients may be related to different symptoms with respect to the attitudes toward one's body.

In turn, further studies on measuring psychological traits in various samples of men and women (healthy and suffering from other mental and physical disorders and/or disabilities) will allow to verify the hypotheses on the relationships between psychological traits and various indices of body image distortions, both within and beyond the population of eating disorder patients.

The DSM-V created by the American Psychiatric Association (2013), the five-factor model of healthy personality (Widiger & Costa, 2013), and the hybrid model of psychological diagnosis of personality pathology suggest a multidimensional approach to identifying dysfunctional personality traits, which can often be observed among eating disorder patients. Among significant psychological traits which bear inclusion into the multidimensional model in future psychological studies on eating disorder patients (especially including orthorexia and the anorexic readiness syndrome, both described in this book) are the traits described in the Big Five model and the DSM-V. A dimensional description of the psychological traits listed below would allow for specifying the characteristics of psychological functioning of healthy people who may nevertheless be at higher risk for developing eating disorders. Among the psychological traits in the Big Five model which are worth including in the psychological diagnosis are:

- Agreeableness – allows to assess the distance/closeness in interpersonal relationships.
- Openness to experience – allows to assess the person's distance/motivation toward gathering new experiences.
- Conscientiousness – allows to assess the person's attitude toward responsibilities (high/low).
- Extraversion – allows to assess the need for stimulation (high/low).
- Neuroticism – allows to assess the need psychological resilience or sensitivity toward experienced difficulties.

In sum, further studies on psychological traits in samples of different ages and sexes, both healthy and suffering from various psychosomatic disorders and/or disabilities (including post-surgery disabilities) will allow for a better understanding body image and esteem, and thus, more effective treatment.

The final notable area of further studies involves refinements in measuring multidimensional, sociocultural aspects (mass media messages, peer and family messages) of the so-called westernization syndrome. It is worth pointing to the value of including the universal (irrespective of actual place of residence or upbringing), western cultural media messages about body image norms, first as a predictor of body image development, and as a predictor of eating disorders.

Conclusions

Following the multifactorial model of the development of eating disorders, the author divided the psychosocial factors important for the diagnosis of the body image into three categories: facilitating, triggering, and maintenance factors. It should be noted that, due to the subject matter, Table 8.1 only shows those psychosocial factors that enable the development of basic guidelines for body image diagnosis in eating disorders. Certainly, the diagnosis of biological risk factors is an important element which should also be taken into account, if only to exclude an organic (biological) basis of the disorder in a given patient. However, due to the significant role of psychosocial risk factors for body image distortions indicated in the literature, Table 8.1 presents their summary to clarify the process of psychological diagnosis of patients with eating disorders. Due to their specificity, medical aspects of the diagnosis require a separate study.

The multi-factor model of the psychosocial risk factors for the development of body image distortions in eating disorder patients serves as a guide for focusing on the holistic approach toward a comprehensive (medical and psychological) diagnosis of (somatic and mental) health and the equally holistic and multidimensional (accounting for a range of determinants) psychological treatment of eating disorders. The models of treatment of eating disorders highlight the importance of multidimensional treatment interventions focused on the diagnosis of the determinants and maintenance mechanisms of the disorder (including body image), without strictly focusing on symptom reduction and a narrow, nosological diagnosis based on the current medical classifications. The psychological diagnosis of body image distortions in people with eating disorder, taking into account the psychodynamic diagnosis of personality structure, as well as integrative psychotherapy present the opportunity for using a flexible and evidence-based combination of various techniques in the treatment of body image distortions in various eating disorders. This also highlights the significance of creativity and spontaneity in psychodrama techniques. These constitute psychological variables which play an important role in generating cognitive and emotional insight, providing inspiring knowledge about the patient, and facilitating corrective emotional experiences.

The above results, presented with reference to established psychological theories, including the author's own results based on her clinical experience with treatment of eating disorders, as well as the suggestion of an integrative approach toward the psychological treatment of body image distortions in eating disorders represents only one possible pathway on the journey undertaken by physicians, psychologists, and psychotherapists toward treating various self-destructive symptoms of anorexia, bulimia, and binge eating disorder, as well as the increasingly common anorexic readiness and bigorexia, with its related specific (overly intense) readiness to overfocus on the need to possess an idealized muscle mass. The integrative use of group and individual psychodynamic psychotherapies together with psychodrama techniques in the treatment of eating disorders may constitute an important pro-health prognosis for the entirety of the comprehensive process of treatment of body image distortions in eating disorders.

References

American Psychological Association (2006). APA Presidential Task Force on evidence-based practice. (2006). Evidence-based practice in psychology. *American Psychologist, 61*(4), 271–285.

American Psychiatric Association (2013). Diagnostic and statistical manual of mental disorders (5th ed). ISBN 10:0890425558.

Clarkin, J. F., Fonagy, P., & Gabbard, G. O. (2013). *Psychoterapia psychodynamiczna zaburzeń osobowości* [*Psychodynamic psychotherapy of personality disorders*]. Wydawnictwo Uniwersytetu Jagiellońskiego.

Lingiardi, V., & McWilliams, N. (2019). *PDM 2 Podręcznik diagnozy psychodynamicznej.* Tom 1 [Psychodynamic diagnostic manual (2nd ed., Vol. 1)]. Wydawnictwo Uniwersytetu Jagiellońskiego.

Widiger, T. A., & Costa, P. T. (2013). *Personality disorders and the Five-Factor Model of personality.* American Psychological Association.

Index

Locators in **bold** refer to tables and those in *italics* to figures.

For Product Safety Concerns and Information please contact our EU
representative GPSR@taylorandfrancis.com
Taylor & Francis Verlag GmbH, Kaufingerstraße 24, 80331 München, Germany

www.ingramcontent.com/pod-product-compliance
Lightning Source LLC
Chambersburg PA
CBHW060316220326
41598CB00027B/4343

9 7 8 1 0 3 2 1 6 9 4 8 4